Organic Voice Disorders

Prentice-Hall Foundations of Speech Pathology Series

PRENTICE-HALL INTERNATIONAL, INC., *London*
PRENTICE-HALL OF AUSTRALIA, PTY., LTD., *Sydney*
PRENTICE-HALL OF CANADA, LTD., *Toronto*
PRENTICE-HALL OF INDIA PRIVATE LIMITED, *New Delhi*
PRENTICE-HALL OF JAPAN, INC., *Tokyo*

Organic Voice Disorders

G. Paul Moore

Professor and Chairman
Department of Speech
University of Florida

Prentice-Hall, Inc., *Englewood Cliffs, N.J.*

Library of Congress Catalog Card No.: 72-135024

Current printing (last digit):

10 9 8 7 6 5 4 3 2

Printed in the United States of America
13-640888-5

editor's note

THE SET OF VOLUMES WHICH CONSTITUTES THE *Foundations of Speech Pathology Series* is designed to serve as the nucleus of a professional library, both for students of speech pathology and audiology and for the practicing clinician. Each individual text in the series is written by an author whose authority has long been recognized in his field. Each author has done his utmost to provide the basic information concerning the speech or hearing disorders covered in his book. Our new profession needs new tools, good ones, to be used not once but many times. The flood of new information already upon us requires organization if it is to be assimilated and if it is to help us solve the many different professional problems which beset us. This series provides that essential organization.

One of the unifying and outstanding features of all the volumes in this series is the use of search items. In addition to providing the core of information concerning his subject, each author has indicated clearly other sources having significance for the topic being discussed. The reader is urged to explore, to search, and to discover—and the trails are charted. In so rapidly changing a profession as ours, we cannot afford to remain content with what we have been taught. We must learn to continue learning.

Although each individual volume in this series is complete unto itself, the instructor should welcome the opportunity presented by the *Foundations of Speech Pathology Series* to combine several volumes to form the basic structure of the course he teaches. They may also be used as collateral readings. These short but comprehensive books give the instructor a thoroughly flexible teaching tool. But the primary aim of the authors of these texts has been the creation of a basic library for all of our students and professional workers. In this series we have sought to provide a common fund of knowledge to help unify and serve our new profession.

preface

ACTORS, SINGERS, LECTURERS, TEACHERS, LAWYERS, AND OTHER PROFES-sional users of voice, fear vocal disorders as a primary threat to their economic and social welfare. Otolaryngologists, pediatricians, neurologists, psychiatrists, psychologists, and speech pathologists see voice defects as a major challenge to the science and art of rehabilitation. Many speech pathologists and others concerned with vocal therapy are reluctant to work with voice problems because they believe their education and training have not prepared them adequately for that responsibility. This attitude is widespread, despite the venerable age of vocal reeducation as a specialty and the existence of a substantial bibliography. The limited assistance for voice disorders that now exists is lamentable, and increased attention to these problems is needed. Perhaps this book can contribute to the field, and it is this hope that constitutes the primary justification for its presentation.

The focus of the material is on voice disorders that are caused by alteration of the organs that produce voice. This special attention does not imply greater importance of problems with organic bases than those arising from functional causes; it simply acknowledges the fact that voice defects are complex enough to require attention to both organic and functional causes. The book stresses certain fundamentals of phonatory theory, as well as etiology, diagnosis, and therapy for vocal disorders, but it is not a self-help manual, and it is not addressed to the beginner in speech pathology. It assumes that the student and practicing clinician have been introduced previously to the field of speech disorders and to the area of voice deviations among the complex collection of communication problems.

The content of the book is based upon both direct clinical experience with voice disorders and laboratory study of normal and abnormal laryngeal function. Much is yet to be learned, but there is encouraging evidence of accelerated research on vocal disorders and on the processes of phonation in laboratories in several parts of the world. As basic information accumulates, it will contribute to the fundamental premise of this book, which is that rational therapy for voice disorders must be based, whenever possible, upon experimentally confirmed physical and physiological concepts related to both normal and abnormal functioning of the vocal organs.

The very attempt to name and otherwise recognize the many persons who have contributed in some degree to the content and construction of this book is a humbling experience. There is a real indebtedness extending over many years to students who have helped focus the ideas, and to colleagues who have challenged, modified, and added information, both directly and indirectly. In addition, special recognition is due to the National Institutes of Health, particularly the unit now called the National Institute of Neurological Diseases and Stroke, for its substantial support of the research that is basic to much of the theory expressed. I am also pleased to identify the following individuals who have contributed uniquely: William H. Shearer, Ph.D., who prepared the anatomical illustrations in Chapter II; Paul H. Hollinger, M.D. and Hans von Leden, M.D., who made it possible for me to become directly acquainted with certain laryngeal diseases and disorders; the late Clarence T. Simon, Ph.D., who guided me into the study of voice disorders; and Gertrude Conley Moore, who helped in uncountable ways and whose name would   appear on the dedication page if there were one.

G.P.M.

contents

chapter III

chapter IV

chapter V

chapter VI

"PEOPLE TALK TO EACH OTHER." THE IMPLICATIONS OF THIS DECEP-
tively innocent statement permeate every aspect of man's complex
world, including his art of expression and his methods of studying
the processes of that art. When people talk to each other, a cycle of
events is traversed which includes thinking, symbolization of concepts, utterance of language, hearing, and comprehension.

If there is impairment at any stage of the communication sequence, there will be some disorder in the end product. If the disturbance involves the basic sounds of which speech is composed,
in contrast with the sounds of language, a voice disorder is present.
The vocal difference may be in pitch that is too high or too low,
loudness that is too great or too weak, or vocal quality that lacks
excellence by being hoarse (rough) or harsh, or breathy or spas-

1 *voice disorders: a definition*

modic or hypernasal or hyponasal or mixtures of these and other
factors.

Experience has given each individual a definition of the preceding terms, and it has also provided a concept of the normal voice
on which judgments of the abnormal are based. Yet it is obvious
that there is no single sound that can be called "normal voice"; instead, there are childrens' voices, girls' voices, boys' voices, womens'
voices, mens' voices, voices of the aged, and so on. In each of these
types of voice both the normal and the abnormal can be recognized.
The location of the threshold that separates the one from the other
is judged by each listener on the basis of his cultural standards,
education, environment, vocal training, and similar factors, but
wherever the separation between adequate and inadequate is placed,
it is obvious that each individual has acquired concepts of normalcy
and defectiveness. This observation should alert the speech clinician
to the fact that voice disorders are culturally based and socially
determined. A voice judged to be defective by the clinician may be
unnoticed by the employer or teacher. The social and cultural fac- 1

tors provide the basis for defining voice problems as those deviations in pitch, loudness, and quality that are judged to be atypical of the voice characteristics of most persons having the same age, sex, and cultural background.

1 Does the concept of normal and abnormal voice presented by Van Riper and Irwin (88:166–71) differ from that found here?

PHONATION AND RESONANCE

Speaking is a complex, learned process that involves the generation of an undifferentiated sound in the larynx and the modification of that sound in the pharynx, mouth, and nose. The production of the sound is known as phonation, and the modification of the sound is called resonance. Phonation ordinarily is accomplished by the vibration of the vocal folds, but when these parts are missing or cannot function, other structures may substitute as the phonatory mechanism. The three vocal elements, *pitch, loudness,* and *quality,* are individually related more or less directly to phonation. *Pitch* is the auditory correlate of the frequency of vibration of the sound source and consequently is determined almost entirely by the vibrator. *Loudness* is the sensation related to the amplitude of molecular motion in the sound wave. This movement results from the volume-velocity of the glottal air pulse which is created by the interaction of glottal resistance and the force of the breath. Consequently, it may be said that loudness is controlled primarily by the vibrator but varies directly with air pressure. *Quality* is the auditory impression created by the complexity of the sound wave. This complexity is related to the number and strength of the partials that compose the sound, and these in turn are determined by the combination of the vibratory patterns of the sound source and the selective alteration of the sound in the resonators.

PHONATORY DISORDERS—DYSPHONIA

PITCH. If a small child has a pitch level that is noticeably higher or lower than that of most of the other children of the same age in his cultural group, that voice according to definition is defective. It may not be unpleasant to the listener, but it is atypical; it suggests an abnormality that requires diagnostic and possibly therapeutic attention. When an adolescent boy or a man regularly speaks with a vocal pitch that is similar to that normally used by a preadolescent or a female, the pitch is atypical and consequently is judged to be defective. If the pitch of a woman's voice is low enough to sound masculine, it is different from that expected and is customarily classified as abnormal.

Two other forms of pitch deviation are monotony and tremulousness. Some individuals habitually speak with little variation in pitch; their voices do not convey the intended intellectual and emotional content of the utterance. Other persons may have tremulous voices in which the pitch, and sometimes the loudness, fluctuates rapidly and without relation to the meaning being expressed. The degree of abnormality is determined by the extent to which the variation differs from that which is customary.

The vocal pitch deviations to which reference has been made represent the three types of pitch problems that are frequently encountered and which may be generalized as follows: 1) voices that are consistently higher than most of the voices used by other persons of comparable age and sex within a particular cultural group; 2) those voices that are lower in reference to the same circumstances; and 3) voices that do not vary in the customary manner in relation to the speaker's intended meaning.

Abnormalities of pitch establish significant relationships between the individual and his environment. The man with a high-pitched voice who is addressed as "Ma'am" or "Miss" on the telephone is distressingly handicapped in both his economic and social life. In modern America, the pitch of the male voice is related to concepts of masculinity; high pitch is often interpreted as a sign of delayed sexual development or as an evidence of effeminacy. A person with such a voice is apt to be rejected by both men and women, and there are few occupations in which he can obtain employment.

An equally distressing problem exists when a woman's voice has a masculine pitch. Various interpretations of masculinity-femininity confusions are made by laymen, and there are certain jobs that are not available to women with masculine-type voices. However, penalties for low-pitched voices in women do not appear to be as severe as those accompanying the opposite situation in men. Part of this difference may stem from the fact that certain prominent actresses have developed low-pitched voices that tend to be admired and imitated. Another probable reason for the acceptance of low-pitched female voices is that laryngitis and other laryngeal diseases almost always lower the pitch; consequently, the change can be associated with an "honorable" disease instead of with a "suspect" physical condition or personality.

The medical, social, and personality implications of vocal monotony, tremulousness, and inappropriate melody patterns range from neurological disorders to laryngeal disease, social inadequacy, and fear. Except for tremulousness, the layman rarely notices these differences. However, in the latter problem, except as it exists in older persons and those experiencing stress, the social and economic consequences can be extensive.

> 2   The problems designated as "puberphonia" and "androphonia" by
>   Greene (39) add interesting reading.

LOUDNESS. When a voice is either too loud or too quiet in relation to a specific environmental situation or when the loudness variation is inappropriate to the meaning of the utterance, the voice is considered to be defective.

Voices that are too loud or not loud enough are faulty because they do not satisfy the requirements of a specific speaking situation. Yet these problems are rarely classified as defects by the general public. Nevertheless, they may reflect situations of extreme complexity with which the speech pathologist must be familiar and to which he should be alert. Individuals who speak too loudly or too quietly most of the time, rarely do so all of the time; consequently, the vocal aspects are interpreted as evidence of, or symptomatic of, a complex problem which itself needs remedial attention. The person with a loud voice may frequently be recognized by his posture and general behavior as an individual with a hearing loss; his voice is explainable on a socially acceptable basis and there is no social penalty. On the other hand, the person who often speaks loudly as though he were excited or egotistical or angry without obvious cause will be considered odd, and social penalties will result. The individual who speaks too quietly in the classroom or in a social situation and who is not physically weak is considered to be shy or socially retarded. In some social groups, this "quiet voice" is fostered among young women, but it is usually condemned in young men as an evidence of weakness. It is probable, therefore, that appropriate loudness of the voice constitutes one of the principal signs of social competence among educated people.

When atypical loudness of the voice is recognized as a symptom of complex psychological and social factors, its therapy is usually not a primary concern of the speech pathologist. However, when a voice cannot be produced at loudness levels that are adequate for the communication needs of the individual, then training is indicated. Clergymen, statesmen, teachers, and others who address large groups need to be able to speak in a loud voice for extended periods without damaging the vocal organs. Before public address systems were developed, public speakers were required to cultivate voices that could be heard easily in auditoriums and lecture halls. Many of the speakers of the earlier eras trained their speaking voices with as much care and detail as that practiced by concert and opera singers. Now when almost every meeting room and auditorium is equipped with microphones and loudspeakers, voices are not taxed as they once were. Even so, persons in public life who must speak to large groups benefit markedly by learning to use a "big voice"; they speak with less strain and fatigue, they have voices that are more pleasant to hear, and they are less apt to develop laryngeal disorders that are caused by vocal abuse.

INTERRELATIONSHIP OF VOCAL FACTORS. Description and classification of discrete disorders, such as the pitch and loudness deviations presented previously, are simplified for textual presentation, but they tend to obscure the fact that these differences often exist concurrently and may vary in relation to each other. Furthermore, pitch and loudness are often intertwined with other types of speech and voice disorders. The multiplicity of vocal factors and their complex combinations contribute to the varieties of voice and consequently to the difficulty of description and classification. Disordered voices are composed only rarely of single types of deviation; usually they contain mixtures of vocal elements that are themselves variable in degree. An awareness of the audible components of vocal sound and the development of the capacity to recognize them are essential to successful management of voice disorders.

QUALITY. The perception of pitch and loudness occurs early in life, probably because the ear mechanism responds directly and uniquely to the two acoustic factors, frequency and amplitude, that are responsible for these sensations. Evidence of the universality of these auditory sensations is revealed in the geographical distribution and antiquity of tonal scales and musical notation. On the other hand, a third type of auditory sensation, variously labeled "quality," "character," or "timbre," is not associated uniquely with a single dimension of auditory response; this feature is the result of mixtures of frequency and amplitude. There is no musical notation for quality, but an analogy to music will aid in the description of quality as that term relates to voice and voice disorders.

A listener can identify the tones of a trombone, a saxophone, and a violin even when all three are producing sounds at the same pitch and equal loudness. It is also true that a musical instrument sounded by an untrained person may emit tones that contrast painfully with those produced by a skilled musician. Furthermore, trained musicians can purposely cause the same instrument to vary its tonal quality, even when the pitch and loudness levels are held constant. These tonal differences constitute quality or timbre; they result from the number and relative intensities of the component elements of the sound wave, and they differentiate voices just as they do musical instruments.

Everyday experience demonstrates that individuals have distinctive voice qualities, most of which are accepted as normal within the person's cultural and ethnic groups. However, there are also voice qualities within each population group that are considered to be defective. The limits of normalcy are not clearly defined, but it seems that voice quality is classified as defective by educated Americans when it interferes with intelligibility, when it suggests a disease or a physical anomaly, and when it deviates from the normal enough to attract attention to itself. These conditions are not mutually exclusive; in fact, they are interdependent to such an extent that it would be difficult to consider one without involving the others.

Voice quality disorders have been descriptively labeled in the literature as breathy, husky, hoarse, harsh, throaty, metallic, thin, hypernasal, denasal, and so on through a great number of terms. Unfortunately, these labels do not denote the same meanings universally, and their diversity reflects both the complexity of voice problems and the current lack of basic information about voice production. It would be presumptuous at this time to suggest that any one set of terms is superior to another. However, since names are required in an orderly presentation, some arbitrary selection is necessary. The choice in this presentation is based partly on tradition, but, more importantly, each of the terms used to denote one of the dysphonias is associated more or less closely with specific phonatory or resonance phenomena which appear to be linked with the auditory factors that are the voice disorders.

3   What are the terms used by Murphy (71) to designate voice quality disorders?

The term one hears applied frequently to vocal deviations is "hoarseness," a label that usually refers to a group of phonatory disorders that are popularly associated with "laryngitis" or "cold in the throat." Many persons with otherwise normal voices experience hoarseness temporarily during the course of an upper respiratory disease, or intermittently when mucus accumulates on the vocal cords, resulting in a roughness of voice that is relieved when the offending material is removed by coughing or clearing the throat. This personal experience with hoarseness enables individuals to associate the problem with the larynx and to recognize the disorder as phonatory. Hoarseness has a roughness and noisiness about it that contrasts with the smoothness of the normal voice. There are many varieties of hoarse quality and degrees of severity that are complicated additionally by changes of pitch and loudness. It is probable that the countless combinations of these several factors heard in abnormal voices contribute to the jumble of terms that are applied to voice quality deviations.

The commonness of hoarseness reduces its social stigma, yet persistent hoarseness may carry serious implications about health, employability, or social adjustment. Hoarseness always means that the vocal cords are not functioning normally. If the disorder is of recent origin, it may be a symptom of disease or structural change that requires immediate medical attention. On the other hand, if the voice has been hoarse for some time and the laryngeal condition is stable, the health implications become secondary to the social and economic considerations. A hoarse voice may reduce the individual's personal effectiveness by making him difficult to understand or unpleasant to hear and thereby restrict his choice of occupations.

Another term that is associated frequently with voice quality is "breathiness," a problem which, like hoarseness, has many varieties

and degrees of severity. Its name suggests that the important audible component of the sound is the noise that is produced by the
flow of breath, similar to that heard in whispering. The typical
breathy voice is weak and low-pitched, except when the individual
attempts to speak loudly; at this time, the noise of the air often
becomes independently conspicuous and the vocal pitch may slide
upward irregularly out of control. Some voices, particularly those
heard occasionally in obese older persons, may shift rapidly back
and forth between hoarseness and breathiness. Younger persons who
abuse their voices by yelling vigorously, frequently observe a progressive change from normal voice to hoarseness, to breathiness, and
even to aphonia if the larynx is sufficiently traumatized. The alter-
nation between breathiness and hoarseness is a common feature of
many voices, but this fact should not lead to the assumption that
the underlying patterns of vocal cord vibration in these vocal disorders are similar. Subsequent discussion will present the distinctive
characteristics and also indicate why the acoustic shifts can occur
in the same larynx.

> 4   What are some of the variables that affect breathiness that are pre-
>   sented by Moore and Abbott (70:488-89)?

A third quality disorder that can be associated with a distinct
type of laryngeal function may be called "harshness." In the current
literature there are many terms that apparently refer to this type of
vocal deviation and most writers classify the cause as functional.
A common description of this problem states that, "Harsh voice
quality has an unpleasant, rough, rasping sound" (51:203). Van
Riper and Irwin point out that tension in the speaker is one of the
behavioral characteristics associated with harshness and that vocalization is sudden with frequent glottal catches and stops (88:232).
Harshness has been identified by some clinicians as a clinical entity
that is recognized primarily by the presence of a sound often called
"vocal fry" (44). This voice quality is distinctive for its repetitive
popping or ticking sound. The vocal pitch is always extremely low
and the frequency of the pulses that produce the popping characteristic may become slow enough to be heard as separate vocal pops
or ticks. Breath noises are weak or absent with this type of voice,
and it usually cannot be produced loudly or with the normal phonatory breath flow. The characteristic low frequency range of vocal

fry sound and its presence in most voices at the extended low portion of the total vocal range has caused it to be considered by some as a vocal register. If an individual uses this type of voice frequently, it can be classified as functionally deviant in the same sense that persistent use of the falsetto is so classified.

5   Observe how "vocal fry" is described in the article by Hollien and Wendahl (44).

A simple or uncomplicated form of harshness is found commonly in the speech of adolescent boys and young men who attempt to lower the vocal pitch below the normal range in an effort to sound more masculine. It may also be heard in such character stereotypes as the "tough guy," "high pressure businessman," "stage witch," or the quiet "confidential auctioneer." This quality is combined occasionally with hypernasality, which adds to the unpleasantness of the voice and may obscure its basic characteristics. Harshness is usually classified as functional, but the vocal fry type of phonation and the resulting voice may also be caused by laryngeal pathology.

In that type of harshness in which a "rough, rasping sound" predominates, some of the characteristics of hoarseness are also present and may result from pathologic changes in the larynx. Swollen vocal cords or tumors can influence vocal cord vibration and consequently affect the sound that is produced in much the same way that hypertense adjustment of the vocal cords and reduced air flow produce harshness. The frequency of vibration is lowered, greater than normal air pressure is required, and vibration is characterized by an abnormally long glottal closure. The most revealing difference between functional harshness and harshness caused by organic change is the greater persistence of the latter. The functional problem tends to disappear during shouting, laughing, increased breath flow, and general relaxed situations; the quality when caused by pathologic conditions is less variable.

SPASTIC DYSPHONIA. The dysphonias that have been described previously have been phonatory problems in which the continuity of voice has been present at all times. In contrast, spastic dysphonia is characterized by momentary interruption of phonation, which results from sudden, intermittent squeezing of the vocal folds against each other. This interruption of sound occurs commonly on vowels and is most obvious when such sounds occur in the initial position of words.

Speech in spastic dysphonia lacks fluency and has been described as a form of stuttering limited to the larynx. The voiced portions of the speech vary among individuals and from time to time will vary also within the same person. The sound associated with this spasmodic speech may be hoarse or tremulous. When the disorder is serious, it frequently makes the speech almost unintelligible and, consequently, extremely handicapping. The inconsistency of the symptoms has caused it to be labeled frequently in the literature as hysterical dysphonia. However, some experimental work suggests that there may be a neurological cause, and this accounts for its inclusion in the present discussion.

> 6   How tenable is the hypothesis that spastic dysphonia is caused by a
>   neurological disorder? See the discussion by Aronson et al. (3 and 4)
>   and by Robe et al. (79).

The problem is a serious impediment to the person who has it because it limits both employment and social contacts. It is found almost always in adults, but mild symptoms of the disorder have been observed also in several teenage persons.

APHONIA. The absence of vocal sound, *aphonia,* is a disorder in which the individual who is afflicted speaks only in a whisper. The loss of voice can occur at any age but is more common in adults, and it may develop either suddenly or over a period of time. It has been observed that the voices of some patients may vary intermittently between complete aphonia and brief bursts of vocalization, but these symptoms are relatively rare.

Most persons in our society have lost their voices temporarily at some time, either as the result of shouting at an athletic contest or in conjunction with "laryngitis." In consequence, the problem carries no real psychological or social penalty. However, persistent aphonia can signal the presence of serious laryngeal disease or emotional disturbance that must be managed through medical referral. Aphonia as a vocal symptom limits the patient's employment and his association with friends; it can be frustrating and emotionally disturbing. However, its social acceptability makes it an ideal escape from competition and responsibility for those who wish such relief. The range of possible causes for aphonia, from organic impairment to hysterical reactions, emphasizes the importance of careful diagnosis and close cooperation between the medical profession and speech pathology. The speech pathologist usually assumes his rehabilitative role after the physician and surgeon have performed their therapies, but he may have the initial responsibility for evaluation and referral.

RESONANCE PROBLEMS

In the preceding description of voice disorders, the entire emphasis was placed on the larynx and the phonatory deviations originating there. However, as pointed out earlier, when the sound that is generated in the larynx passes through the pharynx, mouth, and nose, it is unavoidably modified by the resonance characteristics of the passageway. As the volume and shape of the respiratory tract are varied, a selective emphasis is exerted on the partials in the complex tones that are flowing through. Such adjustments not only create the vowels and consonants, they also contribute to such paralinguistic factors as individual or personal voice characteristics. When the nasal passageway is opened to the resonance system by the lowering of the soft palate, a so-called nasal component becomes prominent in the sound. This audible element is normal in the [m], [n], and [ŋ] consonants but is abnormal in all other English sounds except in certain regional dialects.

HYPERNASALITY. Hypernasality is a term that includes several voice qualities that are associated with the excessive use of the nasal resonator. When one of these voice deviations is present singly or as the most prominent aspect of a complex voice disorder, the voice is described as being hypernasal, and it may carry serious social and economic consequences for the person who possesses it. In some forms it interferes with the intelligibility of speech; in others it implies defective oral structures or an impoverished cultural background. Usually it is aesthetically unpleasant to hear. Hypernasality is frequently blended with disorders of phonation, thereby creating extremely complex vocal deviations in which the component parts are difficult to identify individually.

Most persons have heard speech which seems to be escaping from the nose of the speaker; some of the consonant sounds are accompanied by nasal snorts, and there is extensive modification in the formation of many sounds. The oral plosives and all sounds that are normally non-nasal become nasalized. This type of hypernasality accompanies those conditions that prevent the closure of the velopharyngeal valve, such as paralyzed velum, cleft palate, or short palate. The disorder is often referred to as *rhinolalia aperta* to indicate that the problem results from a relatively large continuous opening between the oro-pharynx and nasal space.

Another type of hypernasality is called nasal twang and represents a form of voice deviation that is usually functional. It is associated in various forms with certain dialects and with hawker occupations such as auctioneering and newspaper vending. However, a similar sounding voice disorder occasionally accompanies the presence of polyps or other nasal obstructions situated anteriorally in the nose. In this instance, the nasal passage, rather than the mouth, becomes a closed cul-de-sac resonator. The individual necessarily breathes through his mouth, but the velopharyngeal area between the pharynx and nose remains open. The condition has been called *rhinolalia clausa anterior* and presents a dilemma that can trap the hasty diagnostician; the voice has a nasal quality, but the individual cannot breath easily through his nose. The condition can be approximated by pinching the nares and attempting to "talk through the nose."

> 7   The concept of nasality being caused by a *cul-de-sac* deserves detailed study and complete understanding. See West, Ansberry, and Carr (94:196–99, or West and Ansberry (95:104–8), and Van Riper and Irwin (88:242–43). The student should draw sketches of the airway to illustrate the various ways in which the nasal passage may be closed, and the conditions resulting when it is left open.

HYPONASALITY. It is customary in discussions of voice disorders to contrast the lack of normal nasal resonance, hyponasality, with excessive nasal resonance, hypernasality, even though the sounds associated with the two conditions are dissimilar and the underlying causes are different. Hyponasality is the quality that accompanies a "cold in the head" or blockage of the nasopharynx by enlarged adenoids, polyps, or other obstructions. This type of voice disorder is sometimes called *rhinolalia clausa posterior,* in contrast with *rhinolalia clausa anterior,* and suggests the nature of the voice as well as the location of the closure.

The denasal voice can be produced purposely by substituting the

[b], [d], and [g] sounds for the nasal sounds in a sentence such as "spring has come in the mountains" which would then be pronounced, "sprig has cub id thuh boududz." Obviously, the concept of functional disorder applies in this particular instance where the velum is intentionally substituted for a pathological obstruction.

The phonetic character of hyponasality has led some writers to suggest that it be considered an articulatory disorder rather than a voice problem. This point of view can be strongly supported, particularly since the critical modifications in the sounds constitute phonemic differences. It has also been suggested that hypernasality be classified as an articulatory defect since the nasal continuants are substituted for the voiced plosives. However, most of the vocal modifications in hypernasality are not phonemically significant in English and, consequently, have less justification for classification as an articulatory problem.

There is considerable evidence, both in the literature and from direct clinical experience, that hypernasality is audible as a distinctive quality which permeates the speech of those who have the problem. It can be recognized apart from the language sounds being spoken in the same way that hoarseness or breathiness can be heard as entities. A nasal component can be added to all vowels and to all voiced consonants except the nasals; conversely, a denasal component can be added only to the three nasal sounds. Consequently, it is appropriate to treat hypernasality as a voice disorder and to include hyponasality in the consideration on the basis of custom and for convenience of discussion.

However, this controversy is largely academic, since the individual who has hyponasality as the result of a nasal obstruction usually also has phonatory problems that are secondary to the obstruction. Mucosal congestion and excessive mucus lead to hoarseness and thereby create a genuine voice problem, which still relates to the original problem that requires medicinal and possibly surgical treatment.

8   The student should become familiar with the various aspects of the controversy between the phonetic and non-phonetic concepts related to hypo- and hypernasality as presented by Van Riper and Irwin (88:2), and Sherman (82).

MUFFLED VOICE. Some persons have voices that are variously labeled as muffled, throaty, or retracted. The quality can be simulated by speaking when the back of the tongue is retracted into the pharynx as far as possible. Comedians sometimes use a voice of this type when they are representing a "country bumpkin" character. This vocal deviation is probably functional in most cases and suggests a dialectal base, but it is also related in some patients to enlarged lingual tonsils that fill the vallecular space between the back of the tongue and the epiglottis. The tonsillar mass keeps the epiglottis pressed backward toward the posterior pharyngeal wall, thereby constricting the lower pharyngeal area, altering the normal resonance characteristics and, consequently, influencing the voice quality.

FREQUENCY OF VOICE DISORDERS

In a society where a variety of vocal differences are accepted as normal and where vocal abnormality depends upon the judgmental standards of the listener, it is almost impossible to obtain a verifiable number that represents the frequency of voice disorders in the entire population. A recent survey in a large elementary school system indicates that as many as six percent of the students have abnormal voices of some seriousness, but this figure probably cannot be projected to the adult population (*80*). Voice disorders, in contrast with articulatory problems, stuttering, and most other disturbances of speech, often begin in adulthood or do not become evident until adolescence. In fact, it can be presumed on the basis of the development of disabilities of all kinds within the population, that the organic (and psychogenic) disturbances that cause voice deviations are probably more numerous among adults than children. This factor adds to the complexity of vocal pathology, increases the demands upon persons working in the field, and emphasizes the need for close cooperation among allied professional groups.

Voice Disorders and the Speech Pathologist

While it is important to the student and professional worker to have some idea of the number of potential patients, the statistical matters lose significance when an individual confronts his own vocal disability. His needs will not differ if there are half as many or twice as many others with the same disorder. He wants help and finds little solace in the knowledge that there are others with similar problems. Voice disorders, even when they are not grossly evident, may be distressing to the individuals who possess them. These abnormalities may alter professional careers, create serious psychological scars, and warp family relationships. Such problems demand skillful handling by competent speech pathologists working in close association with laryngologists, neurologists, pediatricians, psychologists, and other professional personnel.

MOST ADULTS ARE AWARE, IN A GENERAL WAY, OF THE FUNCTION OF the respiratory tract, through which air flows to and from the lungs. They recognize that this airway is composed of the mouth, nose, pharynx, larynx, trachea, and lungs. Observation and incidental study have revealed that vocal sound is produced when the vocal cords, which are located in the larynx, are set into vibration by the breath during exhalation. Most people have felt the vibration of the vocal cords upon touching their Adam's apple or anterior area of the neck while they were talking. This common information is a valuable reference point when the speech pathologist is called upon to aid an individual who has a voice disorder.

When such a person presents himself to a speech pathologist for help, a professional relationship is established and the clinician is

2   *the mechanism of the voice*

expected to know what to do. The steps would be routine if each voice defect were related directly to a specific structural or functional cause; diagnoses would be unnecessary and therapy could be guided by recipe or computer. It is unfortunate, perhaps, that defects of voice cannot be managed with such precision, but the audible factor, the symptom, does not often reveal its etiology; its possible causes are frequently hidden in heredity, disease, trauma, and surgical alteration. Diagnosis and treatment of organic voice disorders usually involve medical specialists in various fields, and it is not only desirable but necessary to combine the professional skills and information of these related disciplines with speech pathology. However, to do so successfully requires meaningful communication among these specialties, which demands insight and knowledge within each group as well as a common vocabulary. One of the minimal expectations is that the speech clinician understand and be conversant with the anatomy and physiology of the organs used in voice production.

Such knowledge is equally important as a basis for the voice evaluations and therapy carried on by the speech pathologist. Many strange ideas about voice disorders have been constructed on foundations of misinformation, and no one can know the number of errors in therapy that have been practiced because the clinician did not understand the mechanism with which he was working.

Persons who are already familiar with the anatomy and physiology of the vocal organs can use this chapter as a review outline. Those who have not studied in this area should look upon the section as a base from which to explore the detailed literature.

STRUCTURE OF THE LARYNX

Since vocal sound and the phonatory disorders are generated in the larynx, this organ offers an appropriate place to begin a detailed description of the mechanisms of voice production. It will be observed in the subsequent presentations that the larynx has been featured much as is the jewel in a ring; the adjacent supports are independently important, but they are relatively subordinate to the central stone. This focal emphasis results from the subject being discussed and should not imply that the larynx is more important to oral communication than the tongue, soft palate, or any other essential structure.

> 9   Terms will be introduced from time to time which must be in the ready
>   vocabulary of the speech pathologist. It is advisable, therefore, for
>   him to have and to use a medical dictionary. The student is also urged
>   to locate, by palpation and mirror observation, his own vocal structures
>   when possible. He will benefit from reference to Harned (41) and
>   Wood (97).

The larynx is a midline organ located in the anterior part of the neck, immediately deep to the skin and a few thin muscles. It extends approximately from the jaw-neck angle downward to within a short distance above the sternal notch and can be palpated readily. If the finger is placed on the Adam's apple, which is the prominence of the thyroid cartilage, and pushed upward a fraction of an inch, a small v-shaped notch can be felt. This region has no functional significance in phonation but is useful as a reference point for the identification of other structures. It may be seen in Figure 1A and B.

Immediately above the thyroid notch there is a small soft area which is bordered above by what feels like a hard horizontal ridge. This structure is the anterior part of the hyoid bone, a u-shaped member which is represented in the same figure and which is usually considered to be the upper boundary of the larynx.

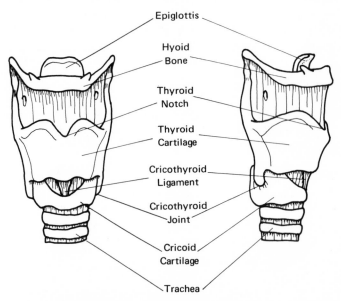

Figure 1. Hyoid bone and cartilages of the larynx. (A) Front view; (B) Lateral view from the right side.

If the finger is moved directly downward from the thyroid notch along the cartilage, a distance of one-half to three-quarters of an inch, another soft area will be felt which is bordered below by another prominent hard ridge. The soft region represents the separation between the lower border of the thyroid cartilage and the upper part of the anterior section of the cricoid cartilage. The lower border of the cricoid ring is designated as the limit of the larynx and also the division between it and the trachea. However, examination of the structures demonstrates that the parts are continuous and indicates why the cricoid cartilage is sometimes referred to as the upper limit of the trachea.

Laryngeal Cartilages

Two of the five major cartilages of the larynx have been encountered in the preceding reference to the external features of the anterior section of the neck. These two, the thyroid and the cricoid, are unpaired midline structures that lie across the median sagittal plane. Another single cartilage that crosses the median plane is the epiglottis. This member is shaped somewhat like a leaf and rests almost vertically above the vocal cords with its stem end attached

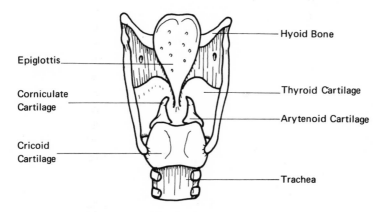

Figure 2. Hyoid bone and laryngeal cartilages: posterior view.

just above the anterior commissure. The two other major cartilages are the arytenoids, which are paired and rest on the cricoid cartilage approximately at the junction of its posterior plate and the lateral portion of its arch. There are also two pairs of minor cartilages, the corniculate and cuneiform, which are unimportant in phonation and consequently will not be discussed here. These structures can be identified in Figures 1 and 2. The student is urged to refer to these illustrations throughout the subsequent discussions.

Since the major cartilages provide the supporting framework of the larynx and its muscle attachments and since the cartilages are functionally important in phonation, it is desirable to examine certain of their features in some detail.

Thyroid Cartilage

The thyroid cartilage is the largest of the group, and although its size varies considerably among individuals in conformity with their other structures, some concept of its dimensions can be gained from the following measurements: the angle formed by the two alae is about 90° in men and up to 120° in women; the vertical midline junction between these wings is about three-quarters of an inch long, and the distance between the line of junction and the posterior border of each ala is approximately one and one-half inches; the vertical dimension of either ala also averages about one and one-half inches along a line in front of the inferior and superior cornua, which, in turn, measure vertically about two inches from tip to tip. These dimensions are given to help those who work with voices to realize the relatively small size of the structures involved. Photographs, drawings, and motion pictures are apt to create distorted concepts for those who do not have an opportunity to dissect or directly observe human anatomical material.

The internal structures of the larynx are enclosed on two sides by the thyroid cartilage, which forms a triangular area that is open posteriorly. This arrangement and the dimensions further reflect the diminutive size of the laryngeal parts and indicate the protection which the thyroid cartilage gives to the interior larynx and airway. On the outer surface of each ala is a low ridge which extends from the base of the superior cornu downward and forward to the lower border. This oblique line provides attachment for certain extrinsic laryngeal muscles which are described below.

Cricoid Cartilage

The cricoid cartilage is partially surrounded by the lower portions of the thyroid cartilage, to which it is attached at joints located at the junction of the inferior cornua of the thyroid and the articular facets on the cricoid. The contacting areas of the cricothyroid joints are relatively flat and usually ovoid, indicating that the cartilages are capable of rotational and some anterior-posterior sliding movements. The location of the articular facets on the cricoid cartilage should be noted in relation to the margins of the cartilages.

The significance of the motions of the two cartilages in relation to each other during phonation is discussed below.

The cricoid cartilage is a ring that completely surrounds the airway at the top of the trachea. It is thick in cross-section, wide posteriorly in the vertical dimension, and narrow anteriorly. It resembles a signet ring, as can be observed in the illustrations. The cricoid facets of the cricoarytenoid joints are located postero-laterally on the upper angular rim of the cricoid cartilage and not on top of the broad posterior plate where they sometimes appear in anatomical illustrations. The joint surfaces are shaped somewhat like the side of a bean with the long dimension following the underlying cartilage. The axis of each facet has been represented in

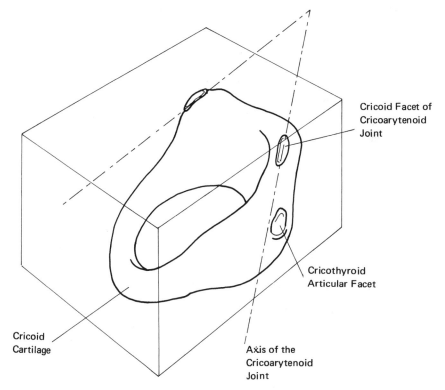

Figure 3. Cricoid cartilage and axes of the cricoarytenoid joints.

Figure 3; it is apparent that the axes extend downward and laterally from a point that is above, medial, and posterior to the facets. The angles of these axes determine the gross movements of the arytenoid cartilages, which are described below.

10   Compare the motions of the arytenoid cartilages as described by von Leden and Moore (90) with those presented by Sullivan, Sauer, and Corrsen (85) and Van Riper and Irwin (88:427).

Arytenoid Cartilages

The arytenoid cartilages rest on the cricoid cartilage at the crico-arytenoid facets mentioned previously. Each of these cartilages has a base and three sides which taper to a peak somewhat like a pyramid. (See Figures 2, 4, and 10.) The posterior face is triangular with the upper angle rising at the medial side; it is concave along its vertical dimension and its surface is smooth. The medial face is also triangular, having its apex curving posteriorly; the surface is relatively flat and smooth. The lower portion of the medial face projects forward in combination with extensions of the base and anterior face to form the vocal process. The frontal or, more accurately, the antero-lateral face, extends from the anterior border of the medial face to the lateral border of the posterior face, somewhat like the widest side of a right angle pyramid. This face has an irregular contour which is distinguished by two large depressions separated by a horizontal ridge. The lower indentation or fovea is identified later as the site of attachments for vocal fold muscles. The arytenoid base, or under surface, is relatively broad and contains a prominent concavity toward its lateral aspect. This depression contains the smooth joint surface that rests on and articulates with the cricoid facet. Immediately beyond the lateral aspect of the arytenoid joint surface, the base of the cartilage terminates in a blunt, rounded projection which is the muscular process. The upper surface of this prominence provides attachment for the lateral and posterior crico-arytenoid muscles. The shape of the arytenoid cartilage gives it great strength at its areas of stress and provides a minimum of size and weight. These factors undoubtedly contribute to the speed and efficiency of cartilage movement which occurs during adduction and abduction associated with protection of the airway and the voicing and unvoicing of sounds in speaking.

Epiglottic Cartilage

The cartilage of the epiglottis is the fifth major cartilage of the laryngeal complex. This structure is shaped somewhat like a leaf, narrow at its stem and widening to a broad rounded extremity. It is attached by a ligament at its narrow end to the inner surface of the thyroid cartilage at the midline, a short distance below the thyroid notch. It projects upward and backward into the pharyngeal area

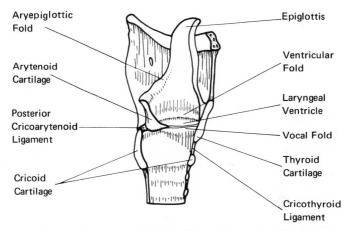

Figure 4. Left half of the larynx viewed from the right side. The structures are exposed by a median sagittal section.

and is supported partly by an elastic ligament extending from its anterior surface to the posterior surface of the body of the hyoid bone. The primary function of the epiglottis is the protection of the airway during swallowing; it helps to close the laryngeal opening into the pharynx and assists in channeling food and water into the esophagus. Since it is relatively unimportant in the production of voice and is not the direct source of voice disorders, it need not be discussed further.

LARYNGEAL LIGAMENTS AND MEMBRANES

Some of the ligaments and membranes of the larynx are important in the functioning of the various parts and consequently contribute to voice production. The moving members of the two laryn-geal joints, cricothyroid and cricoarytenoid, are held in place by ligaments. These bands of tissue maintain the joint surfaces in proper operational relationships to each other and limit motion, thus preventing functional dislocations. Deep to the ligaments, each joint is surrounded by a synovial membrane which supplies and holds the lubricant for the sliding surfaces. The ligaments and membranes of the cricoarytenoid joint are arranged to allow great freedom of motion.

Posterior Cricoarytenoid Ligament

The posterior cricoarytenoid ligament is not directly adjacent to the cricoarytenoid joint, but it is intimately involved with the mo-tion of the arytenoid cartilage. This tissue band extends from the internal face and upper border of the posterior section of the cri-coid cartilage to the lower portions of the posterior face of the arytenoid cartilage. (See Figures 4 and 5). It prevents the arytenoid from sliding too far forward on its facet, and provides a complex radius that regulates the arc of the adductive and abductive motions of the arytenoid cartilages. Furthermore, and perhaps most impor-tantly, it offers an anchorage for the attached arytenoid cartilages when the muscles in the vocal cord contract for phonatory and valvular adjustments. If this posterior anchorage were not present, the contraction of the vocal cord muscles could disarticulate the arytenoid cartilages (90).

Vocal Ligaments

The vocal ligament is a threadlike structure extending from the vocal process of each arytenoid cartilage to an anterior attachment on the inner surface of the thyroid cartilage just lateral to the mid-line. This strand usually parallels the vocalis muscle, supplies sub-stance to the glottal margins of the vocal cords, and probably limits their elongation. The vocal ligament is strongly adherent to the mu-cosal covering of the vocal cords and is formed as the thickened upper border of the conus elasticus. This latter structure is a tough membrane that lies immediately deep to the mucosa in the larynx from the level of the vocal bands down to the lower border of the

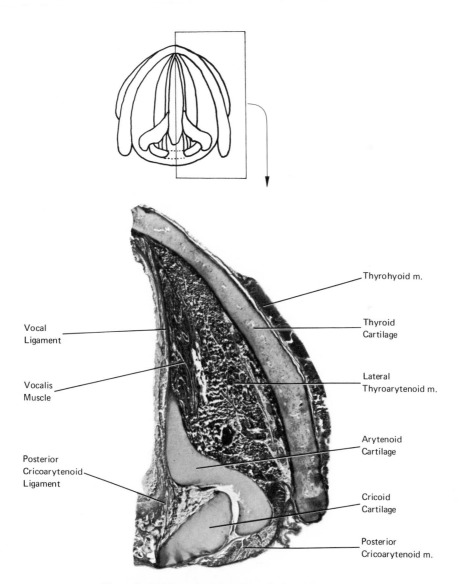

Figure 5. Horizontal section through the right half of the larynx at the level of the vocal ligament.

cricoid cartilage. Anteriorly, in the area between the thyroid and cricoid cartilages, the membrane is continuous with a thickened band called the cricothyroid ligament. The conus elasticus protects the vocal cord muscles from below and may influence vibrational pattern; the anterior ligament limits the separation of the thyroid and cricoid cartilages and indirectly influences the rotational and sliding motions at the cricothyroid joint, which could affect pitch range.

Muscles that support and position the larynx

It is general knowledge that muscles function actively in only one way: they shorten by contraction and consequently tend to draw the structures that are fastened to them toward each other. Since muscles cannot push, there are opposing groups of muscles that draw their associated structures first in one direction and then in another.

Muscles usually are named for the structures to which they are attached, but some are labeled to denote a particular characteristic or position. The student who has not become familiar with anatomical terms will find the names easy to learn if he visualizes each structure clearly and traces the interconnecting tissues.

SUPRAHYOID MUSCLES. All of the bones in the body except one articulate in some manner with other bones; the exception is the hyoid bone situated at the angle of the neck. The larynx is suspended from this bone, which is itself supported by many muscles from the tongue, mandible, pharynx, and skull. However, there are four muscles that operate synergistically to shift the hyoid bone in a forward, upward, or backward direction and consequently contribute importantly to the positioning of the larynx. These are the focus of the immediate discussion.

DIGASTRIC MUSCLE. The digastricus, as the name indicates, is a muscle with two bellies or sections that are joined by an intermediate tendon which is itself attached to the hyoid bone by a sling of connective tissue (Figure 6). The anterior belly runs forward to attach to the inner surface of the mandible near its lower border and slightly lateral to the midline. The posterior belly is longer than its counterpart and extends backward toward the ear to its origin on the mastoid process. Contraction of the anterior belly

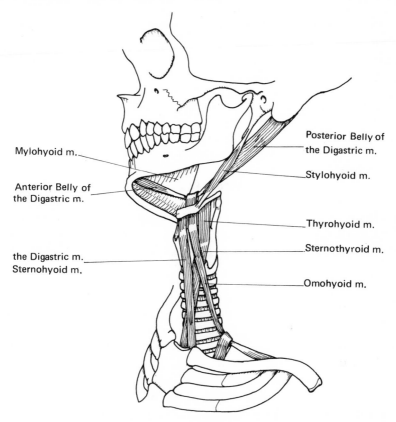

Posterior Belly of
the Digastric m.

Stylohyoid m.

Mylohyoid m.

Anterior Belly of
the Digastric m.

Thyrohyoid m.

Sternothyroid m.

the Digastric m.
Sternohyoid m.

Omohyoid m.

Figure 6. Muscles that support the hyoid bone superiorly and inferiorly.

shifts the hyoid bone forward and upward; contraction of the posterior belly moves the bone backward and upward; when both bellies contract simultaneously, the motion is more or less vertical, depending upon the relative pull from the two sections.

STYLOHYOID MUSCLE. The stylohyoideus is a slender muscle that originates on the styloid process (a bony projection that extends downward from the region of the ear canal) and travels to the anterior portion of the greater cornu of the hyoid bone. Contraction of this muscle lifts and retracts the hyoid.

MYLOHYOID AND GENIOHYOID MUSCLES. The remaining two suprahyoid muscles, the mylohyoideus and the geniohyoideus, arise along

the inner surface of the lower border of the mandible and insert in
the body of the hyoid bone. The mylohyoideus forms the floor of
the mouth, and its posterior fibers tend to lift the hyoid bone. The
geniohyoideus is paired and runs directly from its attachments on
either side of the symphysis of the mandible to the hyoid bone. Its
contraction draws this bone forward.

INFRAHYOID MUSCLES. The muscles which reach the hyoid bone
from below exert a pull in a downward direction. It is evident that
the lifting and shifting by the suprahyoid muscles, combined with a
downward pull from the infrahyoid group, could place the hyoid
bone and the larynx in a variety of positions. There is some clinical
evidence that adjustments in hyoid position are associated with
voice quality and pitch. Whether these modifications contribute to
phonation or simply accompany it is not known at this time, but it
is evident that the problem needs systematic study.

OMOHYOID MUSCLE. The omohyoideus is a long, thin, narrow, two-
bellied muscle that originates along the upper border of the scapula
(shoulder blade) and inserts in the lateral aspect of the body of the
hyoid bone. Between these two attachments the inferior belly extends across the lower part of the neck to the region above the
medial end of the clavicle (collar bone), where it is encased by a
sheath of connective tissue that tethers it to the clavicle and first
rib. The superior belly forms an angle with the inferior section
at the sheath and passes almost vertically to the hyoid bone. The
omohyoideus usually contracts to lower the hyoid at the time of
inhalation, but it is often active during phonation when low pitches
are attempted.

STERNOHYOID MUSCLE. The sternohyoideus is one of the so-called
strap muscles that extend upward from the superior border of the
sternum, or breast bone, along the anterior part of the neck over the
thyroid cartilage to the body of the hyoid bone. The label "strap"
is applied descriptively because the muscles are relatively long, thin,
and of uniform width throughout their length. The descriptive
term is found frequently in the literature dealing with laryngectomy.

STERNOTHYROID MUSCLE. Another strap-like infrahyoid muscle, similar in structure to the sternohyoideus, is the sternothyroideus, which
originates from the cartilage of the first rib and the posterior surface
of the upper part of the sternum. It ascends under the sternohy-

oideus to the thyroid cartilage, where it inserts along the oblique line. Upon contraction it draws the thyroid cartilage downward.

THYROHYOID MUSCLE. A relatively short muscle, having approximately the same width and thickness as the sternothyroideus, extends upward from the oblique line on the lamina of the thyroid cartilage and inserts into the greater horn of the hyoid bone. As might be guessed, it is called the thyrohyoideus. Contraction of this muscle lifts the larynx if the hyoid bone is fixed, or lowers the hyoid bone if the larynx is fixed. The implications of this deceptively simple statement are extremely complex when one contemplates the infinite number of possible adjustments between the suprahyoid muscles and the combined or independent actions of the thyrohyoid, the sternothyroid, and the sternohyoid muscles.

> 11 Some of the infrahyoid muscles are listed in anatomy books as extrinsic
> laryngeal muscles in contrast to intrinsic laryngeal muscles. Which
> muscles in the preceding and following discussions could be classified
> under these terms? See Dorland (27), Ballenger (8:280), or an un-
> abridged dictionary.

INFERIOR PHARYNGEAL CONSTRICTOR MUSCLE. The inferior constrictor muscle of the pharynx is the principal contractile tissue of the lower one-third of the pharynx. This muscle arises from the sides of the cricoid cartilage, the inferior cornua, and posterior areas of the thyroid cartilage. The lower muscle fibers are horizontal and join with the circular fibers of the upper end of the esophagus. This section of the constrictor is sometimes referred to as the cricopharyngeus muscle. The upper fibers of the inferior constrictor become increasingly oblique from below upward as they sweep around both sides of the pharynx to their medial attachments along the posterior pharyngeal wall. Contraction of the inferior constrictor muscle lifts and retracts the larynx to hold it against the posterior surface of the hypopharynx. During swallowing the inferior constrictor relaxes when the suprahyoid muscles draw the larynx forward to enlarge the pharynx. There is some clinical evidence to suggest that persons who appear to exert extreme muscular effort in the neck area and pharynx during speaking are contracting the inferior constrictor muscle and probably most of the other extrinsic muscles also. However, the major reason for the student of voice disorders to understand the role of the inferior constrictor, and particularly that part called the cricopharyngeus, is its relation-

ship to laryngectomy and esophageal speech. This latter group of
muscle fibers often plays an important role in the development of
esophageal voice.

With the exception of the lower fibers of the inferior constrictor,
the extrinsic muscles of the larynx are attached to the thyroid cartilage. This arrangement permits positioning and stabilizing of the
larynx, frees the cricoid cartilage to rotate vertically around a right-
left horizontal axis that passes through the cricothyroid articulations, and, with normal relaxation of the inferior constrictor, the
two cartilages can simultaneously shift anteriorly and posteriorly in
opposition to each other. The significance of these adjustments becomes evident in subsequent discussions of the larynx during phonation.

> 12   How does a laryngologist describe the anatomy of the larynx? A con-
>   cise presentation that will be useful to the speech pathologist has been
>   presented by Ballenger (8:278–84).

Muscles that compose and adjust the vocal folds

The intrinsic laryngeal musculature can be presented more mean-
ingfully when the topography and arrangement of the laryngeal
interior is known. Figure 4 represents the left half of a larynx, as
viewed from the inside, and reveals not only the locations of the
cartilages but also some of the muscles and other structures. In the
upper part of the diagram a vertical, medial section of the epiglottis
is shown, from the lateral border of which the aryepiglottic fold
can be seen extending to its attachment at the arytenoid cartilage.
Anterior to this latter structure, two ridges are shown separated by
a deep recess. The upper ridge marks the ventricular or false vocal
band; the lower represents the true vocal fold or vocal cord; and
the recess denotes the laryngeal ventricle (sometimes called the
ventricle of Morgagni). At the anterior ends of the ventricular and
vocal bands a median sagittal section of the thyroid cartilage is
shown, and below it there appears a section through the anterior
arch of the cricoid cartilage. On the opposite or posterior side of
the airway this same diagram reveals the relative height of the posterior cricoid lamina and demonstrates the placement of the arytenoid cartilage. The lower part of this latter member is below the

upper posterior border of the cricoid cartilage, which demonstrates again that the arytenoid cartilage does not sit upon the signet portion of the cricoid. The location of the arytenoid also indicates the manner in which the posterior cricoarytenoid ligament can secure the arytenoid cartilage to the cricoid cartilage and thereby provide a firm anchor for the muscular contraction of the vocal band.

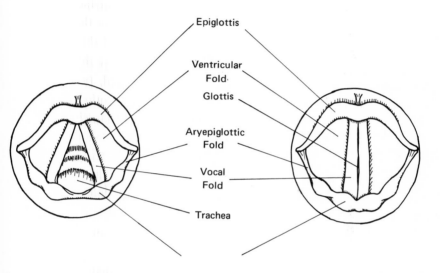

Figure 7. Views of the interior of the larynx as seen from above with the aid of a laryngeal mirror. (A) Vocal folds abducted for respiration; (B) Vocal folds adducted for phonation.

The appearance of the internal laryngeal structures, as seen from above, is represented in Figure 7. For orientation purposes the following structures should be cross referenced in Figures 2 and 4, and visualized clearly for quick recognition: epiglottis, aryepiglottic folds, ventricular folds, vocal folds, glottis, arytenoid cartilages, and trachea.

The intrinsic laryngeal muscles open and close the larynx, adjust the length of the vocal cords, and establish their internal tension and elasticity. (It should be understood that muscle functions of the type indicated are regulated by neural impulses traveling through the nerves attached to the muscles. A subsequent section of this chapter reviews the nerve supply to the larynx.) These functions may combine to form a protective valve to keep food, water, and foreign objects out of the lungs; or they may be synthesized into the delicate adjustments of phonation. The ability of the intrinsic muscles to accomplish these diverse feats is directly related to their size, shape, and location, an account of which is the intent of this immediate presentation. The muscles that will be described are the thyroarytenoid (including the vocalis), lateral cricoarytenoid, two types of interarytenoids, posterior cricoarytenoid, and the cricothyroid.

THYROARYTENOID AND VOCALIS MUSCLES. The mass of muscle fibers that constitute the body of the vocal folds has been described in various ways by different anatomists. Some consider the structure to be a single muscle with two or more parts, while others describe the separate divisions as distinct muscles. For the speech pathologist and teacher the different concepts are not important; the variations that are evident in the literature are pointed out here in an effort to reduce confusion in related reading.

The muscle fibers composing the vocal folds originate on the thyroid cartilage and insert at the arytenoid cartilages. In consequence, they are called the thyroarytenoid muscle or muscles. A medial bundle of fibers that arises from the inner surface of the thyroid cartilage just lateral to the median line and about midway between the upper and lower edges of the cartilage is often designated as the vocalis muscle (Figure 5). This group of fibers, or fasciculus, passes backward parallel with and attached to the vocal ligament and is inserted along the superior and lateral aspects of the vocal process of the arytenoid cartilage. Other muscle bundles originate on the thyroid cartilage beside and below the vocalis along a line that extends downward over the lower half of the thyroid cartilage and onto the upper portion of the central cricothyroid ligament (Figure 8). These fibers pass posteriorly in an upward and lateral direction with the strands that are adjacent to the vocalis inserting on the lower and lateral aspects of the vocal process. Other fibers, originating from above downward, attach progressively along the anterolateral face of the arytenoid, particularly in the inferior fossa. Some of the lateralmost fibers course behind the laryngeal ventricle, and others pass through the ventricular folds to attach to the prominent ridge about half-way up the anterolateral face of the arytenoid cartilage. The muscle fibers in the ventricular fold are designated by some anatomists as the ventricular muscle. Frequently, fibers of the lateral or external thyroarytenoideus also run to the ridge above the muscular process of the arytenoid cartilage and pass beyond as part of the transverse arytenoideus. The length of the thyroarytenoid muscle mass in adult larynges varies from approximately one-half inch in small females to one inch in large males. The rela-

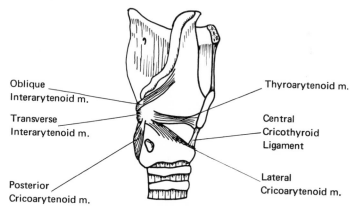

Figure 8. Muscles of adduction and abduction. View of the larynx from the right side with the right ala of the thyroid cartilage removed.

tively small size of the vocal cords makes the complexity of this structure and its function seem even more remarkable.

Contraction of the vocalis and the thyroarytenoid muscles has varying effects, depending upon the positions of the arytenoid cartilages. When these structures, and consequently the vocal folds, are in a lateral or abducted position, they are approximated by contraction of the muscles of the folds. However, when the glottis is closed, additional muscle tension presses the folds together more tightly and also tends to draw the anterior and posterior attachments toward each other, thereby shortening the vocal folds. Activation of the lateral fibers behind the ventricle and the muscle elements of the false vocal folds moves these structures toward the midline to constrict the supraglottic section of the larynx. There is no direct evidence that the vocalis and the thyroarytenoideus operate independently of each other, but the possibility is expressed frequently in the literature and seems to be supported in laryngeal studies. This concept contends that contraction of the lateral portions of the thyroarytenoid muscle shortens the anterior-posterior dimension of the larynx and thereby allows the vocalis to relax and to be shortened passively. This difference of behavior may account for the flaccid appearance of the vocal bands observed in high speed motion pictures when low pitches are being produced. The adjustment of the vocal folds during phonation is described in the following chapter on phonation.

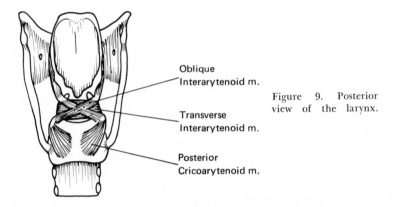

Oblique
Interarytenoid m.

Transverse
Interarytenoid m.

Posterior
Cricoarytenoid m.

Figure 9. Posterior view of the larynx.

LATERAL CRICOARYTENOID MUSCLE. The lateral cricoarytenoid muscle arises along the upper border of the arch of the cricoid cartilage and extends posteriorly to insert into the anterior segment of the muscular process of the arytenoid cartilage (Figure 8). When the arytenoid cartilage is in an adducted position, the pull of the lateral cricoarytenoid muscle almost parallels the axis of the cricoarytenoid joint. In this relationship the force of the muscle is exerted primarily along the axis of the joint to pull the cartilage anteriorly. However, when the arytenoid cartilage is abducted, the muscular process, and hence the muscle attachment, lies farther laterally; consequently, the angle between the muscle and joint axis is greater and the medial component of the muscle action is increased. The combination of the medial and anterior forces creates the possibility of a spiral motion of the arytenoid cartilage on the cricoarytenoid joint. However, the word "possibility" should be stressed because the effects of other muscles, combined with the constraints of the cricoarytenoid ligament, alter the movement in conformity with the kinds of laryngeal behavior needed.

TRANSVERSE ARYTENOID MUSCLE. The transverse interarytenoideus is an unpaired, relatively thick muscle, oval in cross section, that rests in the concavity of the posterior surfaces of the arytenoid cartilages (Figures 8 and 9). It passes from a continuous attachment along the lateral ridge and adjacent face of one arytenoid to similar positions on the other.

Electromyographic investigations have demonstrated that this muscle relaxes during abduction of the vocal folds and contracts during adduction (30). Contraction affects both of the arytenoid cartilages simultaneously and causes each to sweep through a small arc around its cricoarytenoid joint axis and concurrently to slide in a posterio-medial-cranial direction along the joint axis. This combined motion approximates the medial faces of the arytenoid cartilages at the median sagittal plane and consequently adducts the vocal folds.

The action just presented postulates cooperative behavior by the lateral cricoarytenoid and thyroarytenoid muscles previously described. These muscles facilitate adduction and subsequently help both to stabilize the arytenoid cartilages on their joint surfaces and to maintain approximation of the vocal processes.

The lateral cricoarytenoid muscle, in a synergistic relationship with the interarytenoideus, probably also accomplishes the variation in posterior closure of the glottis that occurs with rapid variation of voice pitch. If both lateral cricoarytenoid muscles pull the arytenoid cartilages anterolaterally along the joint axis, the cartilages will separate slightly and the vocal cords will be shortened. These two adjustments appear to occur when the vocal pitch is lowered.

Ultra high speed motion pictures suggest the possibility that the so-called chest register is created in part by loosely approximated arytenoid cartilages that are vibrated by the movements of the membranous portions of the vocal cords. The effect of the additional mass of the cartilages would be a reduction in frequency of the vibrator and a modification of vibratory pattern.

During phonation at the higher vocal pitches the interarytenoideus and lateral cricoarytenoideus hold the medial surfaces of the arytenoid cartilages together tightly and thereby help to provide a firm anchor for the strong contractions of the vocalis and thyroarytenoid muscles. At the same time this tight approximation of the cartilages impedes their vibratory motion and limits phonatory vibration to the membranous portions of the vocal cords.

OBLIQUE ARYTENOID MUSCLE. Some of the adjustments of the arytenoid cartilages that have been associated with the transverse interarytenoideus are aided also by the oblique interarytenoid muscles. These muscles are paired, originate near the muscular processes of both arytenoid cartilages, pass upward and medialward across each other at the midline, and insert near the top of the opposite cartilage (Figure 9). Some fibers continue beyond the upper attachments into the aryepiglottic folds.

The oblique muscles facilitate adduction by drawing the apices of the arytenoid cartilages medially, thereby helping to slide the cartilages around their axes. The direction of pull of these muscles and the mechanical advantage that they obtain by their attachments at the upper ends of the cartilages enable them to exert relatively great power and to move the cartilages rapidly in the closure of the larynx. While the oblique muscles normally function in concert, each acts independently on the cartilage to which it has its apical attachment. This arrangement is in contrast to the single tranverse arytenoid muscle which affects both arytenoid cartilages equally. The capacity for separate functioning of the oblique muscles probably determines some of the adductory motion of the arytenoid cartilage on the healthy side in unilateral paralysis.

The fibers of the oblique interarytenoideus that continue beyond the upper border of the cartilage into the aryepiglottic folds help to pull the epiglottis backward as part of the mechanism of protective laryngeal closure. Concurrently, the aryepiglottic folds are drawn medially as part of the generalized closure pattern.

POSTERIOR CRICOARYTENOID MUSCLE. The intrinsic laryngeal muscles that have been described above close the larynx for phonation and protection of the airway. The posterior cricoarytenoid muscle, which is paired, is the only one that opens the larynx; it is the abductor. Its fibers arise over a broad area on the posterior aspect of the cricoid lamina, extend upward and laterally, as illustrated in Figure 9, and converge to terminate on the lateral part of the muscular process of the arytenoid cartilage. If a plane is drawn through the middle of the muscle parallel to the longest fibers and perpendicular to the muscle mass, it will intersect the axis of the cricoarytenoid joint at an angle of approximately 90 degrees. When the muscle contracts, it draws the muscular process of the arytenoid cartilage around the axis of the joint in a downward and backward direction.

This motion describes a circular arc around the joint axis, at right angles to it, and represents a simple type of rotation. The muscle contraction produces a direct and immediate response of the arytenoid cartilage and undoubtedly accounts for the rapid abduction of the vocal cords. High speed photographs reveal that the glottis can open within small fractions of a second, which provides physiologic support for the common observation that voiced sounds can become unvoiced almost instantaneously. It is probable that the arytenoid cartilage is capable of quicker movement than any other articulated body structure (60).

There are two physical factors that are primarily responsible for the speed and extent of vocal cord abduction that deserve recognition. First, the posterior cricoarytenoid muscle is attached to the muscular process of the arytenoid cartilage close to the joint facet which serves as the fulcrum of cartilage movement. Second, it is the largest intrinsic laryngeal muscle and is relatively quite powerful. Since the arytenoid cartilage approximates a lever and fulcrum system, it is appropriate to apply the principles of such systems to the motions of the cartilage. It is well known that a small movement of the shorter arm of a lever will produce a proportionately larger motion in the longer arm. It is also true that the force exerted at the end of the shorter arm must be proportionately greater to move a load than the force applied at the end of the longer arm. When these principles are associated with the arytenoid cartilages, it can be said that a strong muscle acting on the arytenoid cartilage close to its fulcrum will produce a large motion at the vocal process, which is at the end of the longer arm of the lever. The physiologic effect of this mechanical system is a quick, wide opening of the airway resulting from a powerful short-stroke contraction of the posterior cricoarytenoid muscle.

The primary movements of the arytenoid cartilages are represented in Figure 10 by views of an animated model photographed simultaneously from the front and above. Part A shows the arytenoid cartilages in an abducted position; Part B is a multiple exposure that demonstrates the excursion of these cartilages. The upper image

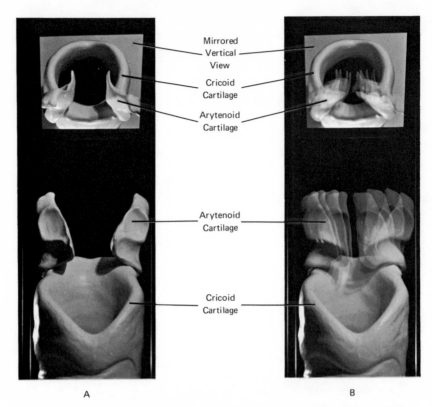

Figure 10. Motions of the arytenoid cartilages illustrated by photographs of an animated model. The upper images are mirrored views of the cricoid and arytenoid cartilages shown below. (A) Arytenoid cartilages in an abducted position; (B) Multiple exposures to illustrate excursions of arytenoid cartilages.

in both parts of the figure is a vertical view, obtained by reflection in a mirror comparable to a laryngeal mirror placed in the pharynx. The movements of the arytenoid cartilages presented in the preceding paragraphs differ in several respects from the descriptions found in many of the textbooks of anatomy and speech pathology. These works describe a rotation of the arytenoids around a vertical axis combined with a horizontal sliding motion toward and away from the glottis. Several investigators (*90*) have demonstrated conclusively that a vertical axis of the type described does not exist and that the gliding motions occur in the direction of the joint axis with a maximum excursion of 2–3 mm. The preceding discussion attempted to present the concepts of the research cited.

THE CRICOTHYROID MUSCLE. It will be recalled from previous descriptions that the thyroid and cricoid cartilages articulate with sliding and rotatory motions at the cricothyroid joints. The muscles that are responsible for these movements are the cricothyroids and their antagonists, the thyroarytenoids, that compose the vocal cords. The cricothyroid muscles are paired and each one has two segments,

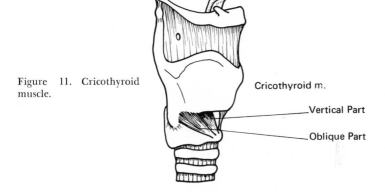

Figure 11. Cricothyroid muscle.

Cricothyroid m.

Vertical Part

Oblique Part

both of which arise on the outer surface of the cricoid ring along the arch and forward nearly to the midline. One segment passes backward to the front edge of the inferior cornua of the thyroid cartilage; the other sends fibers in a more vertical direction to insert along the margin and lower inner face of the thyroid cartilage (Figure 11). Contraction of the more horizontal fibers tends to pull the inferior cornua forward and the cricoid ring backward, thereby sliding the cartilages in opposite directions and increasing the distance between the inner surface of the thyroid cartilage and the arytenoid cartilages, an adjustment that elongates the vocal folds. Activation of the more vertically placed segment of the muscle draws the cricoid and thyroid cartilages toward each other anteriorly, causing a limited rotation at the cricothyroid articulation. When the thyroid cartilage is being actively supported by the extrinsic muscles, the rotational movement will be confined to the cricoid cartilage. However, if the thyroid and cricoid cartilages are equally free or restricted, their anterior parts will move toward each other uniformly. In either situation the rotary motion increases the anterior-posterior distance in the larynx, thereby elongating the vocal folds, decreasing their cross sectional dimension, and increasing their tension. The audible result of the functional elongation of the vocal folds is a rise of pitch. Since the cricothyroid muscles accomplish this adjustment they are sometimes referred to as the "pitch muscles."

NERVE SUPPLY TO THE LARYNX

Detailed description of the motor and sensory innervation of the larynx can be found in all books on general anatomy, and reading in such literature is strongly recommended for greater clinical insight. Familiarity with the function and distribution of the major nerves to the larynx is basic to an understanding of laryngeal performance and disease. The brief sketch presented in the following paragraphs is intended as an introduction and focuses on the superior laryngeal and the recurrent laryngeal nerves, both of which are paired and supply structures on their respective right and left sides.

Superior Laryngeal Nerve

The superior laryngeal nerve branches from the vagus nerve (X cranial nerve) high in the neck, passes downward close to the carotid artery (in which the pulse can be felt at the side of the neck just back of the larynx), and subdivides into internal and external branches at a point a little above the level of the hyoid bone. The internal portion, which is sensory, enters the larynx through the membrane between the hyoid bone and the thyroid cartilage, after which it branches profusely to supply sensory fibers to glands and membranes of the epiglottis and interior of the larynx.

The external branch of the superior laryngeal nerve continues downward along the outside of the larynx to provide motor fibers to the cricothyroid muscle and to the lower section of the inferior pharyngeal constrictor, sometimes designated as the cricopharyngeus muscle.

Recurrent Laryngeal Nerve

After giving off the superior laryngeal nerves, the vagus nerve continues downward through the neck, supplying branches to many structures. When the nerve on the right side reaches the base of the neck, it crosses the subclavian artery where the right inferior or recurrent nerve emerges.

This recurrent nerve loops posteriorly around the subclavian artery, where it encounters the esophagus and trachea which it follows upward to the larynx. On the left side the vagus nerve passes downward to the level of the aorta (just above the heart) before giving off its recurrent laryngeal branch, which swings around the artery posteriorly and passes beside the esophagus and trachea to the larynx.

Both recurrent nerves enter the larynx just posterior to the inferior cornua of the thyroid cartilage and proliferate motor fibers to all of the intrinsic muscles except the cricothyroid. Recent research reveals that the density of nerve endings on the intrinsic laryngeal muscles is quite great, being second only to that of the eye muscles. The implication is that the laryngeal musculature is capable of almost the same order of speed and adjustment as the muscles of the eye (53).

> 13   Observe the histological and electromyographical approaches to the function of the intrinsic laryngeal muscles in (53) and (60).

The pathways and attachments of the laryngeal nerves have clinical significance in both diagnosis and rehabilitation of certain voice disorders. The longer course of the left recurrent nerve into the thoracic area subjects it to greater hazards, and its location in the region of the heart may also account for greater involvement of the left side of the larynx. It has been observed that some phonatory distress is often the first evidence of a circulatory problem.

> 14   The courses of the recurrent laryngeal nerves must be clearly visualized to understand the significance of their locations. Trace them out in Ballenger (8:392–93) or Lederer (55:630–31) or Gray (38:986–92).

RESPIRATORY STRUCTURES RELATED TO VOICE

Professional interest in training and rehabilitation of speech requires a constant alertness to signs and symptoms that may relate to a particular disorder. It is presumed that the student who has completed basic work and is beginning the detailed study of specific disorders has a working knowledge of the structures comprising the respiratory tract. However, experience has demonstrated that some reemphasis of the mechanisms and their functions as they relate to the specific disorders is appropriate. The varied and subtle organic deviations that may underlie voice problems stress the need for sensitivity to every variation from the normal, and, by implication, this requires a familiarity with all aspects of the basic normal.

Air-flow through the larynx is necessary for the production of vocal sound; the breath sets the vocal cords into vibration, and this process creates a series of pressure waves in the air which are heard as sounds. The importance of air-stream to phonation makes it necessary for persons working with voice to understand the basic structures of respiration and their functions.

The fundamental principle of air motion that pertains to breathing is that air flows from regions of higher pressure toward areas of lower pressure. Air pressure may be decreased by expanding its container and increased by compressing the container. When the principle is applied to the thorax, it is evident that as the chest cavity is enlarged, air pressure inside is decreased, and if there are no obstructions, air will flow in; by reversing the process, contraction of the thorax increases the intrathorasic pressure, causing exhalation. The means by which these changes in thorasic volume and air pressure are accomplished constitute the focus of this section.

The Trachea

Previous statements associated the larynx with the trachea, which extends from the cricoid cartilage into the thorax toward the lungs. It is the tube through which the air travels during both inhalation and exhalation. The trachea is held open by a series of closely spaced u-shaped cartilages spaced along this membranous tube. The open sections of the tracheal cartilages point toward the back and provide a flexible posterior wall that lies adjacent to the esophagus. At the lower end of the trachea, which is about four inches long in adults, there is a bifurcation into a right and a left bronchus, both of which continue to subdivide into bronchial tubes within the confines of the lungs until the airway eventually terminates in bronchioles and alveoli, where the gaseous interchanges with the blood take place. The lung spaces expand and contract with the ebb and flow of the air, but they have no power within themselves beyond their elasticity to move the air. Respiration is accomplished

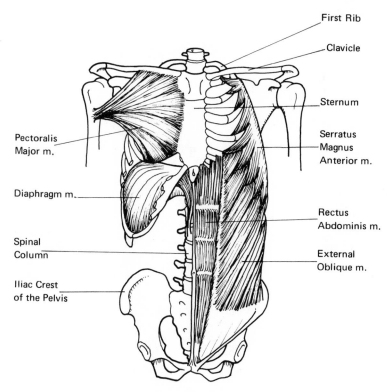

Figure 12. Muscles of respiration.

solely by the radial and vertical expansion and contraction of the thorax.

The Thorax

The thorax, or chest, is somewhat conical in shape, tapering toward the top and is wider from side to side than from front to back (Figures 12 and 13). The walls of the thorax are formed primarily by the twelve pairs of ribs which sweep in a downward direction from the spinal column around the cavity to the front. The ribs are attached posteriorly at joints on the vertebra and by ligamentous connections on the lateral vertebral processes. The significance of the slope of the ribs and the arrangement of the posterior attachment is that the ribs are forced to move outward when they are

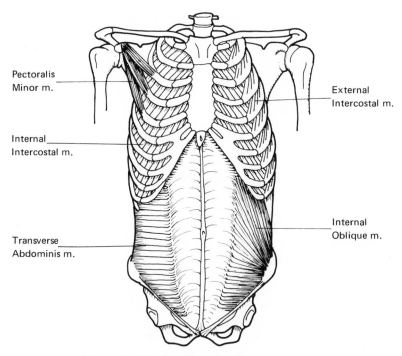

Pectoralis Minor m.

External Intercostal m.

Internal Intercostal m.

Internal Oblique m.

Transverse Abdominis m.

Figure 13. Muscles of respiration.

lifted, which produces a radial-type expansion of the thorax that contributes to inhalation.

The seven upper pairs of ribs are connected individually in front to the sternum, or breast bone, by means of costal cartilages; the next three pairs are attached to cartilages which join similar structures of the ribs above; and the last two, the so-called floating ribs, terminate anteriorly in the muscle walls of the abdomen. The costal cartilages in conjunction with the posterior joints permit rib movements and general flexibility of the chest wall.

The ribs are raised and lowered by several sets of muscles, some of which extend from one rib to another while others connect a rib to an external structure. The muscles that lie between the ribs extend from the lower border of one to the upper border of the one below and are organized into two groupings called the external and internal intercostal muscles. The fibers of the external muscles extend in a downward and forward direction; the internal fibers travel downward and backward. Another intrinsic muscle, the triangularis sterni, extends vertically across several ribs and the sternum on the inner surface of the thorax. External muscles attach the ribs to the vertebrae, to the bones and ligaments of the neck and shoulder region, and to the iliac crest of the pelvis and associated ligaments. The extrinsic muscles include the costal elevators, the subcostals, the superior and inferior posterior serratus, the major and minor pectoralis, the anterior serratus, the latissimus dorsi, and the quadratus lumborum. A clear visualization of their locations and functions is helpful in voice therapy, but since the mechanism of breathing has been described so completely and clearly in other books and since the length of this presentation must be limited, a detailed discussion of the parts of the breathing mechanism and their function has been omitted. Reference is made later to paralysis and laryngectomy, which are the organic conditions that most frequently alter breathing and thereby influence voice adversely.

15   What do Van Riper and Irwin (88:331–46) say about respiration and breathing exercises for speech?

The Diaphragm and Abdominal Muscles

The floor of the thorax is the diaphragm, a musculotendenous partition between the thorax and abdominal cavity that bulges upward, forming an irregular dome which is somewhat higher on the right side than on the left. The central part of the diaphragm is a flat tendon with an irregular contour that is pierced by large blood vessels and the esophagus, the latter going to the stomach, situated immediately below the tendon. The peripheral parts of the diaphragm are composed of muscle fibers extending radially in a downward curve from their insertions in the central tendon to their origins, which circle the lower internal wall of the thorax. The attachments of the diaphragm are located in front on the xiphoid process of the sternum, at the sides on the lower six ribs, and posteriorly on aponeurotic arches and ligaments that connect with the spinal column and posterior ribs. When the muscle fibers contract, they draw the diaphragm downward, thereby enlarging the thoracic area in a vertical direction. However, the actual movement of the diaphragm is more complex than that just implied; the excursions of parts of the central tendon are limited by its attachments to the pericardium and esophagus, thereby causing the major movements of the diaphragm to be lateralized. Furthermore, the posterior muscle fibers are longer and their insertions are lower than those of the other fibers, and consequently the effective motion of the diaphragm is downward and forward. This movement does not alter the fact of vertical expansion of the thorax with contraction of the diaphragm, but it does account for the concurrent forward bulge of the abdominal wall: the diaphragm displaces the content of the viscera downward and forward.

It is this last fact that enables the abdominal muscles to function in opposition to the diaphragm. The coordinated contraction of the four principal abdominal muscles (the external oblique, internal oblique, transverse, and rectus) compresses the viscera, causing it to press against all the abdominal surfaces, including the diaphragm. If the fibers of the latter are relaxed, the visceral pressure will push the diaphragm upward to decrease the thoracic area, increase the internal pressure, and force the air out.

16   A careful study of Fisher's description of breathing for vocalization is strongly recommended (32:40–53).

THE PHARYNX AND VELO-PHARYNGEAL CLOSURE

As the breath is exhaled and the vocal folds are set into vibration, the air and sound flow from the larynx into the pharynx, an irregular tubular space that is shared by both the respiratory and alimentary tracts. The pharynx extends from the esophagus below to the nasal cavities and is continuous not only with those channels, but also with the larynx, mouth, and eustachean tubes. In its lower two-thirds, the pharynx is capable of great change of dimension from front to back and from side to side, a factor that contributes to the act of swallowing and influences vocal resonance. The pharynx is divided into three functional sections that are from above downward: nasopharynx, oropharynx, and laryngopharynx. The nasopharynx reaches from the posterior end of the nasal passages to the level of the palate; the oropharynx extends to the hyoid bone; and the laryngopharynx continues to the esophagus, which begins at the lower border of the cricoid cartilage.

The soft palate and its associated structures are contiguous with the pharynx, and since they contribute importantly to certain organic voice disorders, the region of the pharynx and velum are discussed here in their functional continuity.

The Muscles of the Pharynx

The muscles of the pharynx serve three major functions: (1) transporting and propelling food and liquid to the esophagus; (2) maintaining an airway to the larynx; and (3) regulating the size and shape of the pharyngeal area for phonemic and voice quality resonances. The six muscles of the pharynx include the superior, middle, and inferior constrictors, the stylopharyngeus, the salpingopharyngeus, and the palatopharyngeus. The three constrictor muscles surround the pharyngeal space and constitute the principal substance of the walls of the pharynx. The other three pairs of pharyngeal muscles run more or less vertically, and although they help the constrictor muscles to vary the dimensions of the lower part of the pharynx, their primary function is the lifting of the larynx and hypopharynx.

17 It is essential that the location of the pharyngeal and palatal muscles be known. Almost all textbooks on diseases of the ear, nose, and throat, and general anatomies, have useful illustrations. However, Lederer (55:489–90) and Gray (38:1246–50) present these muscles with particular clarity.

The inferior constrictor muscle was introduced earlier in the discussion of the extrinsic muscles of the larynx, where its several attachments to the thyroid and cricoid cartilages were mentioned. The middle constrictor also has multiple originating attachments that include the lesser and greater horns of the hyoid bone, the stylohyoid ligament, and, minimally, the tongue. The fibers spread fanlike backward and medially around the pharynx to meet their opposite members and to insert along the median raphe that lies anterior to the cervical portion of the vertebral column. The lower border of the muscle overlaps and rests in front of the superior portion of the inferior constrictor, while the upper border, which is approximately at the level of the palate, lies behind the lower fibers of the superior constrictor. The multiple origins of this latter muscle are located on the alveolar process of the mandible, the pterygomandibular raphe, the lower part of the posterior border of the medial pterygoid plate, and among the muscles of the soft palate. The superior constrictor muscle follows the general contour of its fellows and inserts along the median raphe of the pharynx. The upper fibers extend into the nasopharynx almost to the base of the skull.

The stylopharyngeus muscle arises on the styloid process just above the origin of the stylohyoid muscle and travels downward in the lateral wall of the pharynx to terminate among the fibers of the inferior constrictor muscle and on the posterior border of the thyroid cartilage.

The salpingopharyngeus muscle originates from the cartilage of the auditory tube near its pharyngeal orifice and passes downward in the lateral wall of the pharynx, where it attaches among the inferior constrictor muscle fibers along with part of the pharyngo-palatal muscle. This latter muscle also sends some fascicles to the posterior border of the thyroid cartilage in company with fibers from the stylopharyngeus.

The pharyngopalatal muscle is appropriately considered to be a part of the soft palate, but since it terminates in the pharynx, it is equally part of that structure. This arrangement emphasizes both the continuity of body structure and the arbitrariness of the divisions that have been established to simplify description and study.

The Muscles of the Soft Palate

The soft palate, or palatal velum, is a complex muscular structure containing five muscles, two of which have their origins above the palate, two are attached below the palate, and the remaining muscle, which is unpaired, lies completely within the palate, where it extends from its origin on the posterior border of the hard palate to its termination in the uvula. The two muscles that travel superiorly are the palatal elevator and palatal tensor; those that project downward are the glossopalatal and pharyngopalatal. The elevator and tensor muscles and the uvular muscle function synergistically to close the pharyngeal space at the junction of the nasal and oral portions of the pharynx; the glossopalatal and pharyngopalatal muscles oppose the former and contribute to other adjustments described below (38:1246).

The pharyngopalatal muscle (also frequently called the palato-pharyngeus) passes upward in the lateral wall of the pharynx from its attachments on the thyroid cartilage and among the fibers of the inferior pharyngeal constrictor muscle, to its insertion in the soft palate. The palatopharyngeus muscle, with its overlying mucous membrane, forms the pharyngopalatine arch that is often called the posterior pillar of the fauces. It can be seen by looking into the mouth and is recognized as the fold leading from the palate downward and laterally behind the palatine tonsil. The muscle terminates (or arises) near the midline of the velum and forms much of the body of that structure. When the palatopharyngeus muscle contracts, it draws the soft palate downward to open the velopharyngeal valve, an action that occurs rapidly in the production of nasal sounds during speech.

The other palatine muscle that joins the velum from below is the glossopalatinous. It originates on the anterior surface of the soft palate, from where it passes in a downward, forward, and lateral direction to its insertion in the side of the tongue. This muscle is covered by mucous membrane and forms the glossopalatine arch, or the anterior pillar of the fauces, which can be observed as the ridge in front of the palatine tonsil. When the tongue is protruded, it draws the anterior pillar forward and makes it more prominent. If the "ng" sound is produced while the tongue is extended, the glossopalatine arches can be seen to grasp the sides of the tongue tightly to provide posterior closure of the mouth.

The palatal elevator and the palatal tensor muscles, as their names indicate, lift and tense the velum. The former originates at both the cartilage of the auditory tube and the temporal bone, from which it passes downward to the upper medio-lateral surface of the palate, where the fibers spread posteriorly and medially to join those of the opposite side.

The palatal tensor arises from the auditory tube also and from several somewhat scattered locations on the bones of the skull, from which it descends to the base of the medial pterygoid lamina. At this point it attaches to a tendon that passes around a small bony projection, the hamular process, and continues medially to its insertions in the palatine aponeurosis and posteriolateral part of the palatine bone.

The elevator and tensor muscles normally function in concert with the uvular muscle and the superior pharyngeal constrictor to produce the velopharyngeal closure. The elevator draws the palatal structure upward and backward toward the posterior pharyngeal wall, while the simultaneous contraction of the tensor distributes the lift of the elevators throughout the velum and prevents peaking of the palate where the elevators enter the structure. The uvular muscle shortens the uvula and produces a slight bulging of muscle tissue in the central area of contact between the velum and posterior pharyngeal wall, thereby contributing to the closure. It is probable also that the contraction of the uvular muscle increases the tautness of the velum by pulling against the elevators and tensors. The superior pharyngeal constrictor contributes to the valving action by drawing the lateral walls of the pharynx medially. When the closure is viewed from above, its sphincteric nature is evident, particularly at the sides where the puckering is prominent.

NERVE SUPPLY TO THE MUSCLES OF THE PHARYNX AND PALATAL VELUM

The sensory and motor innervations of the pharynx and soft palate involve four of the twelve pairs of cranial nerves: trigeminal (nerve V); glossopharyngeal (nerve IX); vagus (nerve X); and accessory (nerve XI). Each one branches complexly and all are intermingled through ganglia and common nerve trunks, but even rudimentary knowledge of this multiple network can provide clinical insight into certain patterns of disability and sensory involvement. For example, tickling one or both external ear canals will often produce a cough, and, conversely, sharp pain in an ear may indicate the presence of a tumor or infection in the larynx. Such associations can be diagnostically significant to the person working with voice disorders. The four great cranial nerves referred to previously travel to many structures, and their contributions to voice production may be insignificant compared to their life functions, but the special objective of this book necessarily focuses the discussion on the relationship of these nerves to voice disorders. This apparent distortion of emphasis should be recognized as such and not interpreted as myopia of speech pathology.

The trigeminal nerve (V), as part of its distribution, supplies sensory fibers to the mucosa of the mouth, including the soft palate, and sends a motor nerve to the palatal tensor muscle. It also carries some of the sensory fibers to the external auditory meatus.

The glossopharyngeal nerve (IX), as indicated by its name, is associated primarily with the tongue and pharynx. It is composed almost entirely of sensory fibers, but it also carries motor fibers to the stylopharyngeus muscle.

The vagus nerve (X) was mentioned in the previous discussion of the larynx, at which time it was associated nonspecifically with other structures in the neck and thorax. This great wandering nerve also sends sensory connections to the external ear canal and to the pharyngeal constrictor muscles by way of various ganglial connections with the glossopharyngeal nerve. It is probable that the sensory affiliation of the external auditory canal and the larynx is the structural basis for the cough and pain relationships mentioned above.

The earlier reference to the vagus nerve indicated that it was the source of the motor connections to the laryngeal muscles. This is true, but the accessory (XI) which is a motor nerve, gives off many fibers to the vagus nerve at a connection high in the neck, and it is these that branch to the larynx. The accessory nerve also sends motor fibers by way of the pharyngeal branch of the vagus to the pharyngeal constrictors, the palatal elevators, and the uvular muscle.

The complex nerve supply to the pharynx and velum can be summarized and simplified by indicating that the sensory or afferent impulses are carried primarily by nerves V and IX, while the efferent impulses are supplied by nerves X and XI.

The cartilages, muscles, bones, and nerves that compose the mechanisms used in the process of phonation, breathing, and resonation have been described from the point of view of communication. Little has been said about the larynx as a valve protecting the lungs or about respiration as a basic life process or about the role of the pharynx and its associated structures in swallowing. However, it is evident that these biological functions are performed and that the mechanisms used are shared with the communication function. The biological types of activity are primarily reflexive and intuitive; the communication functions are almost entirely learned. This dual use presents very few conflicts and instead demonstrates the responsiveness and adaptability of the structures involved. These characteristics indicate that the processes are subject to modification and learning, a fact that is basic in vocal rehabilitation and training.   ᷦᷦᷦ

PHONATION IS THE PROCESS OF PRODUCING VOCAL SOUND. THERE ARE many variations in this behavior and consequently many kinds of voice. A person may speak loudly or quietly, at a high or low pitch, with a clear or hoarse voice, or he may produce vocal sounds that express anger, exhaustion, skepticism, exhilaration, or any of the other attitudes and emotions conveyed by voice. Each of these vocal characteristics is composed of various combinations of the many sound elements that can be produced in the larynx and resonated in the respiratory tract.

The customary textbook account of the process of voice production describes the breath flowing up the trachea to the approximated vocal folds, where the air pressure increases until it pushes the folds apart, thereby releasing a jet of air which lowers the sub-

3 *the physiology of phonation*

glottal pressure and allows the folds to close the airway. When the breath pressure again increases enough to open the glottis, the cycle of events is repeated and will continue so long as the air pressure and vocal fold resistance maintain their alternating relationship. The series of air pulses created by the periodic interruptions of the air stream generates a sound having a pitch that is directly related to the frequency of the pulses and a loudness that is determined by the amplitude of the sound pressure wave produced.

This description is adequate for the person who needs to know only the general principles of phonation, but it is incomplete. There are several other kinds of phonation that occur regularly in normal speaking and there are additional variations that cause certain vocal defects. The clinician who must attempt to modify laryngeal behavior to affect improvement of a defective voice is required to understand both normal and abnormal phonation as completely as possible. Such information is basic to effective voice therapy.

Phonation is a vibratory process that depends upon the interactions of airflow, air pressure, and an elastic valve. If an engineer   *53* were confronted by problems about such physical factors and their relationships, he would try to solve the unknowns by applying the basic principles that pertain to them. He would observe the composite function as completely as possible and then attempt to consider the influence of each element involved, such as force, resistance, displacement, compression, velocity, and other factors that might contribute to the actions of the total system. If he could not experiment with the natural mechanism, he would construct either theoretical or real models that simulate the elements present, and he would systematically examine the effect of each variable upon the action of all. It is recognized that the larynx and its associated mechanisms are more complex and capable of greater variation than any analagous artificial oscillator and also that there are many unknown quantities in laryngeal behavior. However, there is sufficient information to provide a base for postulations about both normal and abnormal functions. Therefore, it seems appropriate that the speech pathologist emulate the methods of the engineer in an attempt to understand the factors in phonation, even though quantitative measures can rarely be employed.

The study of phonatory anatomy, observation of laryngeal functioning, and analysis of continuous speech demonstrate that the normal mechanism, as well as any model that might be used to illustrate the several features of voice production, must include an air supply that can be varied in pressure and quantity, and a valve that can, when desired, (1) limit the flow of air without oscillation of its parts; (2) momentarily close the airway without producing sound; (3) permit the continuous passage of air while concurrently allowing vibration of the valve elements and the generation of sound; and (4) interrupt the flow of air intermittently and regularly, thereby producing trains of pulsations that initiate sound. Persons who are familiar with the composition of speech recognize that the four kinds of valvular performance just described are related respectively to unvoiced sounds, glottal stops, aspirate phonation, and normal vocal sound.

BASIC FACTORS IN VIBRATION

The forces that must be present to cause vibration in a complex system of the type mentioned include air pressure and elasticity, the second of which is dependently related to length, mass, and compliance of the movable elements. If each of these factors were varied systematically, its effect upon vibration could be assessed and its influence upon phonation inferred. The following review of a few of the basic concepts that pertain to the several variables provides a foundation for understanding the mechanical and dynamic elements that are present in the phonatory process.

Air Flow and Pressure

A constriction placed in a tube through which air is flowing increases the pressure of the air on the supply side of the obstruction in direct relation to the degree of resistance to the flow. It follows that as the orifice in the obstruction is made smaller, the volume of air that can flow through in a limited time is reduced and the velocity of air moving through the opening is increased. When complete occlusion occurs, the pressure against the obstruction and all other boundaries of the supply channel increases uniformly until either the pressure reaches its maximum and the system is stabilized or the resistance is overcome and the air escapes with a subsequent reduction in pressure. Since air and water follow essentially the same laws within the conditions postulated, an illustration of the forces involved can be observed in the valvular adjustment of an ordinary nozzle of a garden hose. As the aperture is constricted, the amount of water flowing is reduced but the stream travels farther, thereby demonstrating greater velocity.

An increase in the velocity of air passing through a tube with a narrowed section reduces the radial pressure along the walls in the area of the constriction. This phenomenon is referred to as the "Bernoulli effect." The theory postulates that the more rapidly a gas or fluid flows through a section of a tube having a reduced diameter, the smaller the lateral pressure against the sides of the constricted part of the channel. Consequently, if the walls of the narrow section are flexible, they will move inward toward each other when the velocity increases, and with sufficient flow they will completely occlude the channel. However, since the Bernoulli effect is present only during motion of the gas or fluid, it will cease when the flow stops. Subsequently, the aperture will be reopened by increased pressure, and if a high velocity of flow again occurs, closure will be repeated. Under appropriate conditions of air pressure and velocity in a flexible channel, a continuous oscillation of the walls can be established. Current aerodynamic theory of phonation postulates that vibration of the vocal folds is caused by a combination of subglottal air pressure and the Bernoulli effect (*33*).

18   What are the two conflicting theories of vocal fold vibration van den Berg discusses (*86*)?

Stiffness and Elasticity

A fundamental characteristic of elastic structures is that each has more or less tension or stiffness, a feature that is evident both in resistance to displacement and the tendency of the object to return to its position of rest following displacement. Resistance to movement and speed of recovery are both directly proportional to stiffness and tension. This principle is illustrated in the response of glass, which is more elastic than rubber; and in the latter, which is more elastic than soft clay. Similar principles of resistance to displacement and speed of recovery are present in a string that can be placed under various degrees of tension (*10*).

Length

When two elastic structures that are the same in all respects except length are set to vibrating at their natural rates, the longer one will take a greater time to traverse its sequence of movements and return to its original position. That is, the longer of the two has a lower frequency, or rate of vibration, than the shorter. This characteristic of oscillation is illustrated visually by the motion of longer and shorter pendulums and auditorily by the pitch of the sounds produced by longer and shorter strings on a piano.

A tensed string that is struck or plucked to one side will not reverse its motion until the displacement created travels to its attachments and is reflected back along its length. Therefore, a relatively wide separation between the supports of a string requires a longer time for the displacement wave to travel to them and back again than when the supports are closer together, that is, when the string is shorter. Consequently, a long string, requiring increased time for the transport of the wave, vibrates at a lower frequency.

Mass

Newton's third law of motion, as applied to the present discussion, could be restated to say: A greater force is required to start and to stop a large mass than is needed to influence a smaller one. The principle involved can be illustrated by contrasting the forces that are needed to roll or to stop a bowling ball and a marble.

19   See Newton's Laws of Motion in an encyclopedia, such as (29).

Compliance

Vibrators that are not uniformly elastic from surface to center, or from one surface area to another, have variable compliance to forces acting upon them. Consequently, regions of greater compliance, that is, areas with less resistance to displacement due to such factors as shape, density of material, or regional flaccidity, are more compliant and will yield to pressure sooner than areas having less compliance.

The relationships between the five concepts just reviewed and the four types of laryngeal or valvular function mentioned previously can be noted in the following descriptions of these latter functions. The way the five basic factors influence vibration, and consequently the sound produced, should be understood by the speech pathologist because the differences between abnormal and normal phonation focus in the vibratory process.

AIR FLOW WITHOUT VIBRATION

When the flexible parts of a model, or the vocal folds, are used specifically as a valve to regulate the flow of air, they do not vibrate and consequently no phonated sound is produced. It might appear that further consideration of this function is unnecessary here since the general focus is upon sound production. However, there are three important reasons for understanding conditions in which vibration does not occur: first, to recognize the forces that can normally prevent such motion; second, to associate the absence of vocal sound with the normal unvoiced elements in ordinary utterance; and third, to provide a foundation for the physiological aspects of aphonia.

The basic problem is to determine the factors that must be present to prevent the vibration of the vocal folds while they are located in any of the possible positions between maximum abduction and complete adduction. It can be presumed that vibration will not occur when the resistance to displacement is greater than the activating forces. This condition could be established in a model by the addition of weights, by increasing the stiffness (elasticity) of the vibrators, by some external interference with their motion, or by preventing the activating force from being effective. This reference to vibratory limiters in a model forecasts consideration of some of the influences that tumors and other diseases might exert on vocal cord vibration.

Persons familiar with the phonetic aspects of speech know that unvoiced sounds are scattered generously through most languages and that these sounds are defined as phonemes in which phonation does not occur. The study of laryngeal behavior shown in high speed films of unvoiced-voice phoneme groups and in fiber optic motion pictures by M. Sawashima and H. Hirose of continuous speech permits the inference that there are two kinds of vocal fold adjustment through which unvoicing seems to be accomplished: (1) changes in elasticity resulting from antagonistic muscle contraction of an isotonic type; and (2) positioning of the vocal folds laterally, out of the force of the air stream.

In the normal larynx the elasticity of the vocal cords can be increased simply by the opposing actions of the thyroarytenoid muscles and their antagonists, the cricothyroid muscles. The former tend to shorten the vocal folds and the latter to elongate them. Consequently, if both groups were to react simultaneously there would be isotonic contraction and a resulting stiffening that could prevent vibration if it exceeded the activating force. The degree of contraction and the consequent stiffness can vary in relation to the air pressure, since the requirement is only that the resistance to displacement be greater than the effective air pressure.

It was pointed out above that the opening of an air channel will reduce the pressure exerted by the enclosed air. Therefore, when the glottis is open, as in abduction, the air pressure against the vocal folds is reduced. So long as the force of the air is less than the resistance in the folds, they will not oscillate and sound pressure pulses will not be generated. It is apparent also that when the vocal folds stop vibrating while they are in a paramedian position, the isotonic contraction is greater than it would need to be if the folds were abducted a greater distance.

Voluntary whispering is a form of speaking in which all sounds are completely unvoiced and represents another example of laryngeal participation in speaking without vocal cord vibration. Observation of normal larynges during the production of whispered sounds reveals that the vocal folds stand either in a slightly abducted position throughout their length, or they are in contact with each other anteriorly and are separated posteriorly primarily between the arytenoid cartilages. These two positionings of the vocal cords have been observed also when phonated sound is produced; consequently, it must be presumed that the absence of vibration during whispering is not caused entirely by the location of the folds in relation to the air stream. Motion pictures suggest that in the abducted position the internal muscle adjustments of the vocal folds create an immobilizing stiffness sufficient to inhibit vibration. In the second position, vibration seems to be prevented partly by longitudinal tension along the vocal folds between the vocal processes and the thyroid attachments. It is also possible that contact between the anterior sections of the folds will at times help prevent vibration.

Whispered speech is produced without vocal cord vibration, yet it is audible. It is composed of sound that is associated with the flow of air; therefore, there must be an air-activated sound source in which some type of vibration occurs. The generation of the "whisper" sound involves some of the principles of air flow and pressure that were discussed previously. When air is forced through an orifice at relatively high velocity, as it is in whispering, and when the surrounding structures are stiff enough to inhibit the Bernoulli response, the air forms a jet that becomes turbulent a short distance beyond the aperture. The turbulence is, in effect, a random vibrator that creates pressure changes in the air that are heard as noise. This type of sound is present regularly in unvoiced consonants, in aspirate initiation of vowels, and in whispering.

When whispered speech is involuntary, it is recognized as a voice defect and is called aphonia. The immobility of the vocal cords that causes the disorder may result from a variety of conditions, including an internal lesion that stiffens them, a tumor on one fold that impinges upon the other and holds both motionless, an interarytenoid tumor or other disease that prevents sufficient adduction to allow activation by the air stream, or some other problem that creates excessive bilateral stiffness. When involuntary whispering cannot be related to an organic problem, the disorder is called hysterical aphonia, and the immobility of the vocal folds results from those types of adjustments that are present when whispering is voluntary. It should be noted that aphonia occurs only when both vocal folds are immobile; if one is capable of vibrating, phonatory sound will be produced.

INTERRUPTION OF AIR FLOW WITHOUT VIBRATION

Unvoiced intervals in speaking also occur when the glottis is momentarily closed by the pressure of the vocal folds against each other. This type of laryngeal adjustment can be observed in photographs of the production of glottal stop sounds. Ultra high speed motion pictures * reveal an essential massive contact between the folds that closes the glottis and prevents vibration. The films also show other laryngeal adjustments that are related to the types of sound that immediately precede and follow the glottal closure.

When a normal voiced sound, such as a vowel, terminates in a glottal stop [ɛʔ], the vocal folds, which are vibrating in an approximated position, are squeezed together progressively during the few diminishing terminal vibrations until motion stops. At this point the glottis is tightly closed and often becomes obscured from view momentarily by the approximation of the ventricular folds. In contrast, when an unvoiced sound such as [h] terminates in a glottal stop, the vocal folds are adducted rapidly during the [h] sequence by the movements of the arytenoid cartilages, which smash together forcefully. The folds do not vibrate during approximation, and after their contact they continue their intercordal pressure as they do when a vowel sound leads into a glottal stop, as described above.

The complex changes that occur during the moment when a glot-

---

* The high speed motion pictures to which reference is made throughout this discussion were produced by the author and his laboratory associates. The photographic rates ordinarily used were between 4000 and 5000 pictures per second, which, when projected, provide ultra slow motion representation of vocal fold vibration (69).

tal stop becomes a plosive and initiates subsequent voiced sounds, are composed of laryngeal adjustments that appear to reverse the movements that are present at the beginning of a glottal stop. The ventricular folds recede rapidly, the pressure between the true folds decreases, and vibration begins with small, constricted glottal openings. The initial vibratory separation between the folds usually starts near the central area of the membranous portion of the folds and extends along only a small segment of the glottis. Each succeeding vibratory opening becomes progressively longer until the vocal folds are active throughout their length. This transition from closure to normal vibration may occur within three or four cycles, or it may require twenty or more, depending upon such factors as the tightness of the glottal occlusion and the rapidity of the shift to the following sound.

When a glottal stop-plosive initiates an unvoiced sound, the first adjustments are similar to those described for a voiced sound. However, the release of the glottal closure is accompanied by the abduction of the arytenoid cartilages and the vocal folds. The latter do not vibrate and ordinarily swing wide to open the airway.

Vibration without glottal closure

Vocal folds may be located permanently or be adjusted functionally in any of several rest positions between adduction and wide abduction. While they are in a separated position they can be set into vibration if the relationships between muscle contraction, air pressure, and flow rate are appropriate for disrupting equilibrium. Normally the paired vibrators move with similar amplitudes, at the same frequencies, and with synchronous motion because the air pressure is exerted equally on both and they have approximately equivalent length, mass, elasticity, and compliance. However, the presence of comparable movement should not obscure the fact that each vocal fold is a separate vibrator capable of independent motion. This concept and a representation of the several factors that influence vibration under these circumstances can be visualized by reference to the accompanying illustrations.

Figure 14A pictures a model in which relatively thick elastic bands, analogous to the vocal folds, are stretched between anterior and posterior attachments and are capable of vibrating laterally and medially. These longitudinal strands provide the elasticity factor that is represented as the heavy spring (E) in Figure 14B. The mass of each total vibrator is illustrated as the weight (M) in the same illustration, and compliance is suggested by the small springs (C) in the medial borders of the vibrating elements. In a system of this type vibration begins when a force, such as an accelerating flow of air, exerts just enough pressure to displace the most compliant area of the vibrators.

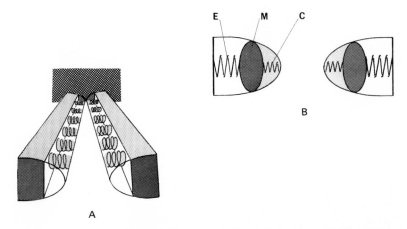

A

B

Figure 14. Model of vibrators separated at one end and capable of motion in medial and lateral directions from their positions of rest. Three factors that influence vibration, elasticity, mass, and compliance are represented in part (B) as E, M, and C respectively.

Ultra slow motion films have revealed that the amplitudes of the initial vibratory movements of abducted vocal folds are extremely small and that the displacement may be limited to a segment of the glottal margin. The first vibratory motion sometimes occurs in a medial direction as the result of the Bernoulli effect; otherwise, the initial movement is lateral, suggesting that the pressure against the folds is greater at that instant than the effect of the flow through the glottis. Initial displacement in a lateral direction will pertain when the edges of the vibrators are relatively thin, a condition that minimizes the factors that are necessary to create the Bernoulli effect. Following the first displacement of the vocal folds in either direction, there is an opposite swing that carries the free margins back through their rest positions and a short distance beyond. This movement is followed by a second excursion that has a slightly larger amplitude in both directions. In each successive vibration the distance traveled increases and more of the mass of the vibrators becomes involved in the motion until a relatively constant condition is established.

Effects of Variation in Air Pressure and Air Flow

After vibration of slightly abducted vocal folds is in process, an increase in air pressure without compensatory adjustments will result in greater amplitude of the vibrators without change of frequency. The vibratory changes are comparable to those that occur in a violin string when a bow is drawn with increasing speed and firmness across the string. The resulting amplitude of vibration is increased but the frequency remains the same.

It should be noted here that the medial phase of the vibratory excursions of abducted vocal folds is often great enough to cause the folds to meet and partially occlude the glottis. Contact may occur only at the anterior portions, but if the amplitude of movement is large, the closure may reach almost to the vocal processes. These progressively variable glottal closures can influence the relative effects of the several factors that determine patterns of vibration and the character of the sounds produced. Some of the discrepancies that have been reported in the literature about the effects of air pressure upon the pitch of the voice may be related to the type and extent of closure in the vibratory cycle. Further discussion of this factor occurs in a later section dealing with vibration having a closed phase.

Vibration without closure causes a sound that is often called "breathy" when it originates in a larynx and "tone mixed with air noise" when it is created by a model vibrator. This complex sound emanates from two types of generators, the air stream itself and the vibrating elements that are activated by the air flow. When the moving members cause the air to pulsate through the intervibrator space in alternately greater and lesser amounts, there are corresponding rhythmic variations in air pressure which create sound waves that are perceived as having pitch. The additional factor in the total sound that is recognized as air noise is caused by turbu-lence in the air stream similar to that present in aspirated sounds and whispering. The mixture of noise coming from turbulence and tone from the action of the vibrators creates the characteristic breathy sound that signals the absence of a closed phase in the vibratory cycle.

An increase in air pressure and flow may be accompanied either by more turbulence and, consequently, a louder air noise compo-nent, or by the reduction of air noise and more audible phonated sound. Greater turbulence will occur when an additional volume of air is forced through an aperture that does not change its size appreciably. Conversely, when the aperture is flexible, an increased air flow will facilitate the medial excursions of the vibrating ele-ments (Bernoulli effect), so that they more nearly close the airway. The resulting effect is greater interruption of the air flow and con-current increase of pressure in the sound pulses which cause a louder tone. This factor may account for the stronger vocal sound that accompanies increased exhalation in some patients who have unilateral vocal fold paralysis.

Effects of Elasticity, Length, and Mass on Vibration without Glottal Closure

When the stiffness or elasticity of vibrators is increased without change in length, a greater activating force is required to establish and maintain vibration. Concurrently, greater elasticity increases the recoil, or restorative force, and causes the vibrator to move toward its rest position more quickly after it has been displaced. Reduced recovery time results in a higher frequency of vibration if the activating force is sufficient to maintain oscillation. Increase of elasticity without change of length can be accomplished in a model, Figure 14A, by replacing one pair of rubber strands with a stiffer set. A comparable modification in elasticity can be accom-plished in the vocal folds by isotonic contraction of the thyroaryte-noid muscles. Greater elasticity of the laryngeal vibrators may also be created by their elongation, which increases their tension.

When the vocal folds are elongated, there is a concurrent reduc-tion in their transverse dimensions and a decrease of the mass at each point along the folds. By application of Newton's third law of motion it is apparent that this modification increases frequency and augments the effect of greater tension. The combined influences of increased elasticity and reduced mass offset the tendency of a longer vibrator to have a lower frequency.

Effects of Compliance on Vibration without Glottal Closure

Compliance is determined in the normal larynx by such factors as varying thickness of the folds between their glottal borders and their lateral boundaries, the tapering width from anterior to posterior attachments, the variable firmness of the internal cordal structures, and the texture of the mucosa. It can be presumed that the area along the glottal margin that is most compliant will yield first to a uniform force such as breath pressure; that is, vibration begins at the area of least resistance. The initial deflection involves only part of the glottis from which the displacement progresses to adjacent areas in successive cycles as vibration develops. This progressive opening undoubtedly contributes to the complexity of the undulations of the folds and probably to the content of the acoustic wave. The amount of curvature of the cordal margins in the undulations seems to be related inversely to the degree of elongation and tension in the folds.

20 Note the discussion of vocal cord motion presented by Leiberman (57) and the related comments (66).

VIBRATION WITH GLOTTAL CLOSURE

When the vocal folds vibrate in an abducted position, as previously described, the movements of their anterior-posterior midpoints trace curves of the type represented in Figure 15A. In contrast, when the folds are adducted, or model vibrators are placed in contact with each other, as in Figure 16A and B, the curves traced by their motions approximate the pattern illustrated in Figure 15B. The vibratory cycle includes lateral and medial movements that are followed by a closed phase which occurs when the vibrators return to and attempt to pass through their positions of rest. The pattern of vibration that contains opening, closing, and closed phases in each regularly repeating cycle customarily represents normal vocal fold vibration.

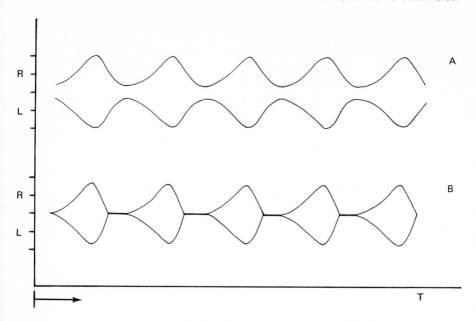

Figure 15. (A) illustrates the lateral and medial vibratory motions at the midpoints of the opposite borders of a pair of vibrators that are separated when at rest. This condition is illustrated in Figure 14. (B) represents the vibratory movements of comparable points when the opposing borders of the vibrators are in contact while at rest. This relationship is presented in Figure 16.

Elasticity, Length, and Mass

When glottal closure occurs during vibration, the variable factors, elasticity, length, and mass, influence frequency and amplitude in approximately the same manner as when vibration occurs without closure. That is, with a constant activating force, greater elasticity produces higher frequency and smaller amplitude; increased mass reduces both frequency and amplitude; and greater length causes lower frequency if the difference in size represents an increase in mass, but if additional length is caused by elongation, the frequency is increased by the consequent greater elasticity and smaller unit mass.

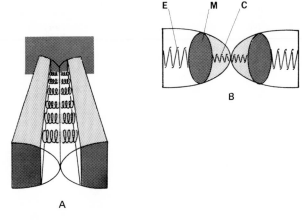

Figure 16. Model of a pair of vibrators that have their opposite borders in contact when at rest. Each unit is capable of lateral and medial motion, but the medial excursion beyond the position of rest is restricted by contact with the opposite member. The factors that regulate vibration, elasticity, mass, and compliance are symbolized as E, M, and C respectively in part (B).

Compliance Factor with Glottal Closure

When paired vibrators do not contact each other, the compliance factor exerts relatively little influence on frequency and amplitude, and contributes only modestly to the contour of movement. In contrast, compliance affects the several variables of vibration significantly when the vibrating elements come into contact with each other. The influence of compliance can be illustrated by picturing adjacent vibrating strings or bars on each of which a steel ball is attached. When such non-compliant, highly elastic elements are drawn in opposite directions and released, they swing together to bounce apart immediately and repeatedly after contact, as suggested by Figure 17. In contrast, if a compliant, less-elastic material, such as sponge rubber, were substituted for the steel balls, the units would be compressed upon impact, and there would be a period of prolonged contact before rebound. The action of a more compliant substance is represented in Figure 18. When this type of reasoning is related to the elements in Figure 16, it is apparent that the degree of compliance represented by the small springs in the contacting areas will contribute to the length of the period of contact; greater compliance causes increased compression and longer closure.

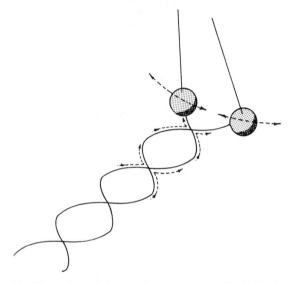

Figure 17. Illustration of the motions of non-compliant, highly elastic substances, such as ivory or steel ball pendulums that are allowed to swing together repeatedly. The units bounce apart immediately after contact.

If the concept of compliance is applied to the vocal folds, it can be presumed that the frequency of vibration, and consequently the pitch of the voice, will be lower when the contacting portions of the folds are softer. Greater compression of the glottal borders is evident in high speed motion pictures when the vocal folds are shortened for lower pitches. This fact suggests that compliance combines with such other factors as mass and elasticity to determine frequency. Further evidence that compliance influences pitch comes from the observation that the vocal sound is lower when the mucosa on the vocal folds is swollen, as is common in such diseases as colds and laryngitis, or when there is edema along the glottal margins.

Compliance also influences the intensity of the sound produced through its effect upon the length of contact between the vibrators and, consequently, on the amount of subglottal air pressure. If two equal amounts of air are released in pulse periods of different lengths, the velocity of air in the shorter pulses will be greater and the sound that is generated will be louder. Similarly, if two different quantities of air are released in time intervals of the same length,

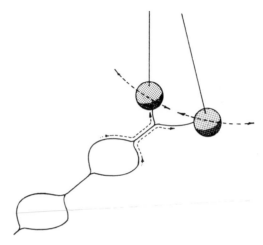

Figure 18. Representation of the reaction of a compliant substance, such as sponge rubber, when pendulums of the substance swing together repeatedly. The pendular units compress each other and remain in contact for a period of time proportional to the degree of compliance.

the larger amount of air will have a greater velocity and, consequently, will produce a louder sound.

21   Note the discussion of volume-velocity by J. L. Flanagan (33).

Compliance in intermittently coupled vibrators of the type being discussed influences not only frequency and intensity, it also contributes to the complexity of vibratory motion and, consequently, to the quality of the sound produced. After two members such as the vocal folds meet each other in a vibratory cycle, the pressure between them continues to increase until their kinetic energy is dissipated. At this point the internal cordal structures begin to move laterally, and the intercord pressure decreases progressively until the elements can be separated again by the air pressure. The time required to accomplish the sequence of change during the period of contact will be determined by a combination of the energy in the vibrators, their compliance, and the activating force that is tending to separate them. The energy that is dissipated while the folds are pressed together can be represented by the dotted lines in Figure 19. If the recession portion of the compression terminates

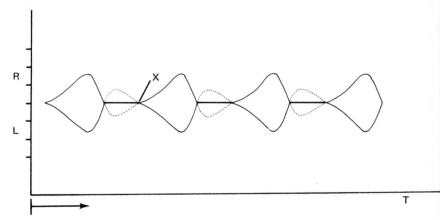

Figure 19. The dotted lines represent the kinetic energy that is dissipated within the vocal folds during the closed phase of the vibratory cycle. The entire pattern suggests that the inter-vocal fold pressure increases and then subsides approximately to that which exists when the folds are in contact and at rest. At that point in the vibratory sequence, which is designated as X, the subglottal pressure is sufficient to open the glottis to start a new cycle. The reciprocal forces that are present create a condition of maximum efficiency.

at the point in the cycle where the air pressure is sufficient to push the folds apart to begin another sequence (Figure 19, point X), the recoil-resonant period of the vibrators and the activating force will facilitate each other to produce maximally efficient vibration. In contrast, if the recoil-resonant period does not correspond with the activating force, the two factors can interfere with each other.

Conflict Between Activating Force and Natural Frequency of Vibration

One possible type of incoordinated response is illustrated in Figure 20. This curve represents the condition in which the activating air pressure is great enough to overcome the medial force during the recoil phase and to separate the vibrators at a non-resonant point. The probable effects of this conflict are a shortening of the closed phase and some modification of the glottal configuration during the vibratory opening.

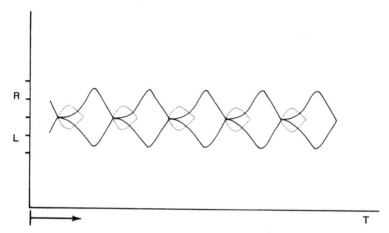

Figure 20. Illustration of a conflict between the activating force and the natural period of vibration. The dotted lines suggest the theoretical concept that the kinetic energy which would normally hold the vocal folds together for a substantial portion of the cycle is overcome by relatively strong subglottal pressure, thereby shortening the closed phase and altering the pattern of motion.

A short closed phase in the vibratory cycle may also occur when there is gentle contact between vibrators and the air flow is relatively great. Under these conditions the folds do not compress each other significantly, and the region that is most compliant will be deflected by the air stream before other areas are disturbed. Consequently, the borders of the vibrators acquire complex curvatures that cause a progressive enlargement of the glottis, which influences both the rate of air release in the glottal pulse and the quality of the sound.

A second type of incoordination between forces is illustrated in Figure 21, which demonstrates a proportionately longer period of contact between the vibrators. Motion of this type occurs when the activating pressure increases relatively slowly to the break-through point. In this situation the recoil-resonant forces are dissipated within the structures before the activating force becomes great enough again to displace them. It is this kind of motion that is present in one type of "vocal fry" phonation.

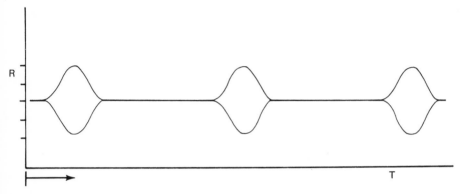

Figure 21. Pattern of vibration associated with "vocal fry," in which the closed phase of the cycle is abnormally long.

Frontal stroboscopic laminagrams suggest that vocal fry may also be produced when the mass of the vibrators is increased by the collaboration of the ventricular folds. These structures appear in x-ray photographs to combine the ventricular folds functionally with the vocal folds to form massive bilateral vibrators that move with relatively small amplitude. It is presumed that this mechanism is capable of both impeding the flow of air, even when there is considerable pressure, and of releasing a series of pulses in which the channel is open for relatively short portions of the cycle.

The principle illustrated in the preceding discussion is that the ratio of open to closed segments of the vibratory cycle in phonation is related to the balance between air pressure and glottal resistance as determined by compliance, mass, and elasticity of the vocal folds. It can be postulated that when the air pressure is relatively large, the glottal opening will be present throughout all or most of the cycle. In contrast, when the resistance is proportionally great, the glottal opening will occupy a shorter portion of each vibratory cycle. High speed films of the vocal folds reveal that there is great variation in the relative length of the three phases of the vibratory cycle. The different patterns of vibration appear to be related to both loudness and quality of sound produced, but at this time the precise relationships are not sufficiently evident to describe.

Asymmetrical Vocal Folds and Vibration

The influences of stiffness, mass, length, and compliance on the motion of paired vibrators that were described previously presumed uniform, symmetrical conditions in both of the moving units. However, since disease and organic changes may not affect both vocal folds in the same way, and since each must be considered as a quasi-independent vibrator, it is necessary to postulate the influence of the several variables when they are altered in only one of the folds.

If the elasticity of one vocal cord were reduced, the following modifications in motion could be expected: The less elastic fold would be displaced before its partner; that is, it would begin its vibratory cycle ahead of the other, its amplitude would be greater, it would tend to have a lower frequency, and its curvature or configuration would be more complex.

If one of the vibrators were weighted more heavily than the other, the heavier member would require more force to displace it; consequently, it would begin to move later than its partner, and its frequency would be reduced. In this type of theoretical consideration it is presumed that other variables remain constant. However, it is recognized that such conditions rarely exist and that, for example, when the weighting of a vocal fold is caused by a tumor, the disease may alter other variables as well.

The cartilagenous framework of the larynx tends to maintain both vocal folds at similar lengths. However, if one of these vibrators were shortened as the result of an injury to the supporting structures, it would become relatively more flaccid and more compliant. Consequently, it would probably respond with less breath pressure, move more slowly, and have greater amplitude than its partner. Conversely, if the shortening were accomplished by scar tissue that reduced the length of the vibrating portion of a fold without changing its mass or elasticity, it would tend to vibrate at a higher frequency and smaller amplitude than the opposite fold.

If one fold, or a segment of a fold, were to become more compliant than the other, the behavior would approximate that associated with change in elasticity. The most compliant area would be displaced first and consequently would influence the shape and progression of the glottal opening. Increased compliance would also contribute to greater amplitude of motion of the more compliant fold and to an asymmetrically shaped glottis.

The deceptively simple sketch of the effects of unilateral differences in mass, length, and compliance just presented should not obscure recognition of the potentially complicated influence of a change of shape of the glottal border of a vocal fold. When a localized protrusion caused by edema or a tumor extends into the glottis, it will influence vibration variously in relation to its size, location, and firmness. Such an enlargement can prevent glottal closure, shorten the vibrational portion of the folds, interfere with the motion of the opposite fold, vary the mass in a circumscribed area, change the elasticity, or modify compliance. The unique set of conditions present in a specific larynx at a particular time will determine the influence of the several factors on pitch, loudness, and quality.

Elevation of One Vocal Fold

In the preceding discussions, both normal and aberrant vocal folds were pictured only in their customary symmetrically opposed positions. This concept is incomplete and needs to be extended to include the condition in which one vocal fold is elevated in relation to the other. This arrangement is not uncommon to a mild degree in otherwise normal larynges and is almost always present in unilateral paralysis. This vertical separation in paralysis is frequently part of the cause of vibration without closure. Displacement of the folds also alters the configuration of the airway and thereby modifies the direction of flow and effective pressure of the air stream. These changes affect the dynamic factors and increase the complexity of the vibratory movements.

22   What are the several changes in the vocal folds that are present with unilateral laryngeal paralysis? See the article by H. von Leden and P. Moore (91).

THE ACOUSTIC SIGNIFICANCE OF ASYMMETRICAL VIBRATION

Earlier statements have emphasized the concept that the vocal folds generate sound through their combined action on the air stream. Typical or normal vibration produces a relatively regular series of pressure waves that are heard as musical tones or smooth sounds. The regularity of sound waves occurs when both vocal cords vibrate at the same frequency and each maintains a relatively regular periodicity.

It has been pointed out that the vocal folds are separate, independent vibrators and that they are capable of moving differently when one is stiffer or heavier or longer or more compliant than the other or when the glottal contour of one differs from that of the other. The vibratory deviations that can occur include different frequencies in each of the folds, greater amplitude of motion in one fold than in the other, phase variations between the motions of the folds, and dissimilar patterns of vibration occurring simultaneously at various segments of the glottis. The first and fourth of these asymmetries usually produce vocal disorders; the second and third have no audible effect on voice so long as the frequencies of both folds remain the same.

The basic premise that pertains to difference in vibratory frequency between the vocal folds can be stated as follows: If the combined action of the individual vibrators creates series of pressure changes in which consecutive waves are randomly irregular in time and/or amplitude, the sound produced will be perceived as rough or hoarse. The upper pair of curves in Figure 22 represent the motions of opposite points on the vocal folds of a woman who had a rough-sounding voice that had been designated as hoarse. It is apparent that one fold vibrated three times while its partner completed only two excursions. These curves also reveal some random variation in both time and amplitude in consecutive vibratory episodes. The combined influence of these two sets of vibrations upon the air stream is represented in the lower curve of the figure. The vertical measurements display the glottal width and suggest a comparable variation in both glottal area and air flow. The random variability of the glottal size also implies a comparable fluctuation in the sound pressure waves and the cause of the rough or hoarse voice.

The critical element in the premise presented in the preceding paragraph is the *random irregularity* in either time or amplitude of consecutive waves (*93*). There are individuals who can volun-

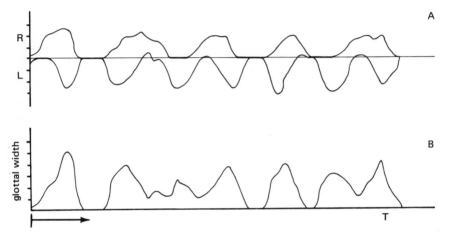

Figure 22. Illustration of vocal fold vibration in which edema on one fold caused a randomly variable vibratory pattern. (A) represents the motions of the right and left folds posterior to the edematous area. (B) demonstrates variations of glottal width and suggests the randomly varying sound pressure pattern responsible for the rough-sounding voice that was produced.

tarily phonate with a different frequency in each vocal fold to produce a double tone. However, these voices are not rough-sounding because each of the cordal vibrations appears to be cyclically regular, and the combined effect of the two sets of movements is a regularly repeating pattern of glottal variation (*92*).

> **23**   Many persons probably are capable of producing diplophonia but have never tried. Read the description of this type of voice as presented by Ward and others (92).

The second type of asymmetrical motions mentioned above refers to those vibratory conditions in which one vocal fold has a wider lateral excursion than the other. The differences in amplitude may be relatively small or they may be maximal, as when one fold is stationary. Figure 23 indicates one example of moderately different amplitudes of motion. Dissimilar amplitudes do not in themselves cause an abnormal voice because the vibrators move synchronously, symmetrically, and regularly at the same frequency to produce a regular train of sound pressure waves. The glottal width curve is

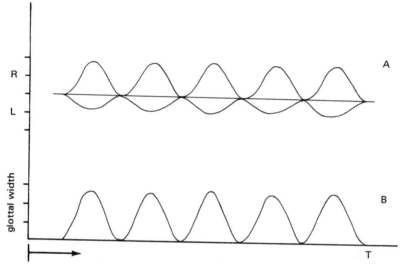

Figure 23. Representation of vocal fold vibration in which the amplitude of movement of one fold was greater than that of the other, while the periodicity remained the same in both. (B) demonstrates the pattern and regularity of glottal openings.

indicated in the lower part of the figure and represents a normal sequence of regular vibratory fluctuations.

"Phase difference," the third type of asymmetry referred to earlier, indicates vibratory motions that begin either at slightly different moments in the vibratory cycles of the two folds or that occur somewhat more slowly on one side than on the other. The example presented in Figure 24 reveals delayed lateral and medial movements for the left fold, but the excursions are regular and create a normal pattern of glottal width variation as represented in section B of the illustration. So long as the phase lag does not cause a change of frequency in one vocal fold, the resulting sound will not be abnormal.

Even though dissimilar amplitudes and phase differences do not generate dysphonia, they are discussed here for two purposes: (1) both of them often appear as abnormal vibratory patterns upon inspection by stroboscopy or high speed photography and they may be associated erroneously with a voice problem, and (2) the abnormal appearance may indicate an organic problem of consequence. Information about the first observation may contribute to the vocal

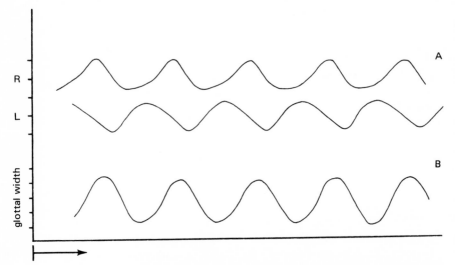

Figure 24. (A) indicates phase differences in the motions of the two vocal folds. (B) represents the pattern and regularity of the glottal openings. The vocal sound produced by this pattern was breathy because glottal closure was incomplete, but there was no roughness in the sound.

diagnosis; knowledge about the second may lead to proper professional referral.

Dissimilar patterns of vibration occurring concurrently at different parts of the glottis are usually caused by a protrusion on the free margin of one vocal fold. The atypical contour of the fold creates abnormalities in vibration in addition to the influences of the increase in mass associated with the protrusion. At lower pitches, when the vocal folds are shorter, more compliant, and vibrate with relatively large amplitude, a protruding area will influence sound generation as follows: As the vocal folds approach each other in the vibratory cycle, the enlarged area will meet the opposite fold and, except for some compressions in both folds, the medial motion at the position of contact will stop. However, the vocal folds on both sides of the protrusion tend to continue their vibratory approximations. Adjacent to the mass there will be no glottal closure, but contact between the folds may occur at some distance away and extend to their anterior and posterior attachments. The air stream will continue its flow in varying amounts through the open areas near the protrusion to create some audible turbulence. The shortened vibrators will release the air pulsations differently from the normal manner to cause a change in the quality. However, the fundamental frequency will not be altered so long as the protruding mass does not remain in contact with the opposite fold throughout the vibratory cycle.

When the vocal folds are elongated for the production of a high pitch, they become more elastic and less compliant than at low pitch. Consequently, when the adjustment for the higher pitch is present, a protruding mass will not be pressed into either the healthy or the host fold as readily when vibratory contact occurs. This condition causes larger glottal openings adjacent to the protrusions and an increase in the air turbulence noise. Furthermore, greater vocal cord tension reduces the amplitude of vibration, and the two folds often remain in contact at the region of enlargement throughout the entire vibratory cycle. This adjustment effectively shortens the active vibrators and causes excessively high pitch. Furthermore, when the protrusion is near the middle of the membranous folds, the glottis is sometimes divided into anterior and posterior sections that vibrate with different frequencies and create double tones. This latter type of phonation usually requires unusually strong air pressure.

The presence of a protruding mass on a vocal fold may also interfere with the vibratory motions in such a way that they are not regularly repetitive. Rates as well as amplitudes may vary randomly and produce corresponding sound waves that are perceived as hoarse or rough sounds. The protruding masses may be confined to the regions between the folds, but occasionally they are more extensive and mobile so that during adduction they slide on top of and rest upon the opposite fold. Such enlarged areas impair the motion of both folds, and frequently they are vibrated somewhat independently by the underlying vocal folds to generate extraneous sounds. The variations and complications are too varied and too complex to permit much generalization.

EXTRANEOUS SOUND SOURCES

Most persons have experienced the temporary vocal effect caused by the accumulation of mucus in the larynx. This secretion collects on the vocal folds and in the glottal space, where it interferes with the usual vibratory movements and acts as a semi-independent vibrator. When it impairs vocal fold motion, it can change frequency unilaterally to contribute to vocal roughness. As a separate vibrator it can be agitated by the movements of the underlying fold and also be fluttered by the air stream. The latter action creates many irregular oscillations of a transient type at relatively high frequency which produce noise. When this kind of vocal problem is present chronically, it suggests either that excessive mucus is present more or less continuously in the larynx or that the mucosa on the folds is loose and capable of being set into rippling or fluttering motions. The essential element in this type of phonatory pattern is the presence of an extraneous vibrator, a sound generator, that is capable of more or less independent, periodic, and sometimes transient oscillation.

Another class of extraneous vibrators includes structures that are not directly associated with the vocal cords, such as the ventricular folds, the epiglottis, and the esophageal sphincter. Ventricular folds vibrate when they are approximated and driven by a sufficiently strong current of air. The behavior of the true folds is obscured from view when the false folds are activated, but there is photographic evidence to indicate that the true folds do not interfere significantly with the flow of air. When ventricular folds vibrate, they are quite aperiodic and thereby generate a sound that is extremely rough. Usually the ventricular folds become active in sound generation only when the true folds are incapable of oscillation.

The epiglottis rarely contributes to sound generation, but this structure has been observed in vibration during the production of voice. The vibratory mechanism is formed by the approximation of the posterior surface of the epiglottis and the structures at the upper portions of the arytenoid cartilages. Sound is produced when the epiglottis moves alternately away from and toward the posterior, superior border of the larynx. The oscillation occurs at a relatively low frequency and results in a breathy, weak, low-pitched sound.

The esophageal sphincter is the mechanism that most commonly generates noise with eructation. When air flows from the stomach, it encounters the closed upper end of the esophagus where, if there is sufficient force and quantity of the air, it forces an opening of the esophageal sphincter. A repetition of the opening and closing creates a sound in much the same manner as that produced at the vocal folds. The essential factor is a mechanism that will emit a series of pressure pulses in the audible frequency range. Usually this eructation, or belching sound, is not used for speaking, but when the larynx has been removed or the vocal folds are unable to vibrate, the esophageal sphincter provides a serviceable phonatory mechanism.

The esophageal voice has a low pitch, it usually is rough sounding, and it frequently contains noise elements. The low pitch and rough sound are caused by the action of the relatively massive sphincter at the junction of the esophagus and hypopharynx. The esophageal lumen is alternately opened and collapsed by the action of esophageal air; the rate is slow and the motion occurs somewhat aperiodically. The extra noise elements are the sounds of air bubbling through liquid. Saliva and mucus always pool in the hypopharynx at the entrance to the esophagus, and as the air escapes in pulses from the esophagus it agitates the accumulated liquid. This bubbling activity creates relatively high pitched noise containing many transients.

The three extraneous vibrators that have been described are observable as distinct entities and have been introduced here to represent various alaryngeal sound sources. However, other sites in the respiratory tract where flexible constrictions can be formed also occasionally serve as sound sources. These include such areas as the fauces and the buccal areas. In the former the tongue is the regulator of the constriction, and the vibrator is either one or both of the posterior pillars or the posterior border of the velum. In the buccal area an air bubble is trapped between the teeth and cheek, then squeezed out, causing the mucosa of the buccal region to vibrate. This sound is moderately serviceable for speech, as Donald Duck has demonstrated.

Vocal Deviations and Organic Abnormalities of the Larynx

Earlier comments have indicated that phonatory disorders include aphonia, in which no vocal cord vibration occurs; breathiness of varying degrees, in which glottal closure is not complete; roughness or hoarseness, caused by random variability in consecutive vibrations; extraneous noise elements which result from the aperiodic (often transient) vibration of mucus, mucous membrane, and other atypical oscillatory structures; and pitch deviations in which vibratory frequencies are abnormally increased or decreased. The kinds of organic abnormalities that are associated with phonatory disorders include paralysis, ankylosis of the cricoarytenoid joints, tumors of various types, surgical or traumatic alteration of structures, scar tissue, and edema or other swellings from local or systemic disorders. The specific manner in which the several organic deviations influence vibration and hence phonation is determined by their size, location, and extent of involvement. However, these organic changes and their attendant deviant vibratory patterns ordinarily do not identify a specific disease or anomaly. It follows that the vocal sound alone is not a reliable indicator of the organic problem. This fact is reemphasized by the observation that voice disorders are rarely composed entirely of one of the types of deviation that are isolated for textbook description. In the real clinical world there is usually a combination of several auditory anomalies. Undoubtedly such blending has contributed to the proliferation of the many descriptive terms that are applied to vocal disorders. Although it is not possible to distinguish specific diseases and alterations of the larynx by the sound of the voice, the character of the vocal sound will reveal much about the kind of vibration occurring and will often provide clues that are vital in the diagnosis of voice disorders. Learning to listen analytically, that is, to dissect the sound, is a great aid in both diagnosis and therapy.

24   Note the recommendations and cautions expressed by Darley (21:56–60).

DISEASE AND OTHER ORGANIC ABNORMALITIES IN THE LARYNX CAN
modify the position, size, shape, mass, mobility, elasticity, and compliance of the vocal folds, thereby causing disordered vibration and
phonatory defects. Disease and organic anomalies can also alter the
resonance spaces of the respiratory tract to the detriment of voice
quality. The speech pathologist is obligated to understand these
organic changes as a basis for effective diagnosis and rational therapeutic procedures. Furthermore, the speech pathologist must be
able to communicate readily with physicians, to comprehend completely the meaning of medical reports, and to cooperate effectively
in the management of patients with vocal disorders. To study the
nature and significance of a disease or the character of a tumor in
no way implies a desire or intention to practice medicine; on the

4 *organic modifications that influence voice*

contrary, such knowledge may help the speech clinician to distinguish more clearly his areas of professional responsibility.

A systematic review of the organic disorders that may cause voice
deviations is presented under the following three headings: (1) diseases that affect gross adjustments of the vocal folds and velopharyngeal valve; (2) localized organic deviations that directly modify
phonation or resonance; and (3) systemic conditions and diseases
that exert their influence on voice indirectly. Such classifications
cannot be completely independent of each other, but they provide
an organization that relates to both diagnosis and therapy.

DISEASES AFFECTING GROSS ADJUSTMENTS

Diseases that affect closure of the glottis and regulations of the
velopharyngeal valve include paralysis, joint disease, and myasthenia.

Paralysis

Paralysis is the lessening or absence of muscle contraction. It usually results from impairment of the nerve supply to the affected structures, but it may be caused also by a local lesion in a muscle, such as a tumor or ulceration, or it may be associated with a general debilitating condition such as a systemic disease or poison. Paralysis may have an almost imperceptible onset followed by a more or less rapid progression. In contrast, it may appear suddenly, or it may occur intermittently, causing changes in both loudness and quality that last over varying periods of time (*40*).

EFFECTS OF LARYNGEAL PARALYSIS. A diagnosis of "unilateral laryngeal paralysis" usually means that the muscles attached to the arytenoid cartilage on the affected side cannot contract and, consequently, the patient is unable to close the glottis. This positioning allows the breath to escape in greater and lesser amounts during phonation in which both folds vibrate without glottal closure to produce a weak, breathy sound. The paralyzed member may be fixed in any position between the median saggital plane and maximum abduction, and it is usually elevated slightly in relation to its healthy mate.

When bilateral laryngeal paralysis exists, both vocal folds frequently rest in paramedian positions, which leaves a narrow glottal airway. This close approximation of the folds provides a relatively efficient vibrator that is capable of producing nearly normal vocal sound. However, the small glottal opening reduces the capacity of the airway, and when the patient increases his demand for breath as the result of even slight exertion, the resulting faster inspiratory flow actually decreases the glottal width through the Bernoulli effect. The result is respiratory embarrassment and threat of suffocation.

IMPLICATIONS OF LARYNGEAL PARALYSIS. Unilateral paralysis is the type that comes most frequently to the attention of the speech clinician and results from impairment of the recurrent laryngeal nerve on the affected side. Frequently the site of the neural lesion and its cause are clearly established by the individual's history and medical diagnosis. These factors may include surgery for the removal of the thyroid gland, other operative procedures in the neck or upper chest, accidental injury to the neck, or specific diseases such as poliomyelitis, diphtheria, or meningitis. However, paralytic involvement of indefinite origin is also common and carries special cautions for the speech pathologist. When the etiology of the disorder is not known, it does not mean that there is no cause; it simply indicates that the diagnostic procedures have not revealed it.

> 25   To obtain a more adequate concept of the large number of causes of paralysis of the larynx, the student should become familiar with the chart presented by Ballenger (8:396–97).

Restoration of normal, or nearly normal, function sometimes occurs without the cause of the disorder being positively identified. However, there are instances of recovery in which subsequent information indicates that viral or other infection was the basic cause. Occasionally, paralysis persists throughout the lifetime of the individual without other change or symptoms. In these cases the presumption is often made that the recurrent laryngeal nerve has been compressed or otherwise permanently damaged. On the other hand, the basic cause of the paralysis may be revealed only after a period of time by the development of additional symptoms. These other signs are commonly associated with such disorders as central nervous system lesions, especially bulbar impairment; circulatory disease, particularly cardiac problems; respiratory disease, primarily conditions involving the upper part of the thorax; tumors in the mediastinum or along the course of one of the recurrent nerves; and toxic effects of either endogenous poisons caused by various diseases, or exogenous poisons such as bromides, iodides, mercury, sulphur, lead, and carbon monoxide.

EFFECTS OF PARALYSIS INVOLVING THE VELOPHARYNGEAL CLOSURE. When either or both of the palatal elevator muscles is paralyzed or when one or both sides of the superior constrictor muscle of the pharynx is similarly affected, a closure of the velopharyngeal port does not occur. Consequently, the nasopharynx and nasal space are continuous with the oropharynx at all times, which creates a constant nasal resonator and a persistent nasal component in the speech. Concurrently, this physiological deviation prevents the increase in oral breath pressure that is necessary for the normal production of plosive and fricative consonants.

The inability to close the velopharyngeal valve also causes difficulty with swallowing. Food and liquids may be squeezed into the nasopharynx by the action of the tongue and non-paralyzed pharyngeal muscles when swallowing is attempted. Persons with this type of paralysis find it difficult to drink from a fountain because the water, after entering the mouth and oropharynx, escapes into the nasopharynx and flows out of the nose.

IMPLICATIONS OF VELOPHARYNGEAL PARALYSIS. The infectious diseases that affect the nerves of the larynx can also influence those that supply the muscles of the velum and pharynx. The involvement may be independent of the larynx, but it is not uncommon to find paralysis of the velopharyngeal muscles accompanying a similar impairment in the laryngeal muscles. This combination is encountered in patients who have had poliomyelitis affecting the neck and indicates involvement of the glossopharyngeal, vagus, and accessory nerves. Persons who have suffered impairment of only the vagus nerve high in its course may also exhibit both palatal and laryngeal disturbances.

When hypernasality of the open type (*rhinolalia aperta*) is present as the result of paralysis, the velum can be observed to behave in one of three ways when vowel sounds are produced. It may hang inertly without positive motion; it may elevate feebly and slowly; or it may swing upward, backward, and laterally. The first reaction suggests extensive bilateral neural involvement; the second indicates partial bilateral paralysis; and the third signals unilateral paralysis on the inactive side. Since congenitally short palate, submucal cleft palate, open cleft palate, and surgically treated cleft palate may also produce hypernasal speech similar to that caused by paralysis, it is essential that the etiologic factors be clearly recognized by the speech clinician.

When a voice disorder is the only, or principal, symptom of laryngeal or velar paralysis, the speech pathologist may be initially and importantly involved with the problem. His awareness of the potential complexities of the basic conditions enables him to enlist medical care for the patient when indicated and to cooperate with the physician in the management of the problem. When the paralysis and voice problem remain as residuals of injury or disease, the speech clinician may occupy the primary rehabilitative role. It is a common observation that when health and survival cease to be the primary concerns of the patient and his physician, the problems of communication become paramount.

Joint Diseases

Inflammatory diseases of various kinds, metabolic disturbances, or constitutional factors that affect one or both of the cricoarytenoid joints may restrict or prevent the motion of the arytenoid cartilages. The condition is believed to be relatively uncommon, but since the adduction and abduction of one or both vocal cords is restricted as in paralysis, the two conditions can be confused. The laryngologist can differentiate between immobility of an arytenoid cartilage caused by paralysis and that resulting from ankylosis of the cricoarytenoid joint by manipulating the cartilage. If it is readily movable, ankylosis has not occurred and paralysis can be presumed to be the cause of the disorder. As would be inferred, the effects on phonation of fixation, or mechanical limitation of the motion of the cartilage, would be similar to those accompanying laryngeal paralysis. When ankylosis has occurred with fixation of the cartilage in a lateral position, the voice is weak and breathy, and the prognosis for improvement through vocal rehabilitation is poor.

Myasthenia Laryngis

Myasthenia literally means a muscle without strength. When myasthenia is present, muscles fatigue quickly with use, and if the condition is present in the larynx, the approximation and adjustments of the vocal folds become less firm and precise as phonation continues. Jackson and Jackson (*46*:313) state that "There are six classes of cases (of myasthenia laryngis) observed clinically; those due to (a) damage of the muscles by violent shouting, shrieking, screaming at football games and other brutal abuses of the larynx; (b) muscular fatigue from prolonged excessive though not violent use; (c) excessive load imposed by a tumor, or an arthritic cricoarytenoid joint; (d) invasion by neighboring inflammatory conditions; (e) general sytemic conditions; and (f) association with chronic laryngitis caused by the abuse." The voice is produced more easily after rest; that is, it is louder and less breathy. The primary signs of myasthenia laryngis that are visible in laryngoscopic examinations are sluggishness of arytenoid movement and the presence of a space between the arytenoid cartilages when adduction for phonation is attempted.

The laryngeal debilities that accompany myasthenia laryngis are similar in their effects on the voice to those associated with the neurogenic paralyses. However, the need for understanding the basic differences between the disorders is essential, since exercises are usually desirable in therapy for paralyses but are contraindicated in myasthenia laryngis until the basic problem is under control.

LOCALIZED ORGANIC LESIONS AFFECTING VOICE

Deviations in the larynx that affect voice include tumors of various kinds, certain infectious diseases, trauma, local irritations, and surgical procedures. Comparable organic deviations may also alter the size and patency of the resonators and, consequently, influence the quality of the sound emitted.

Tumors

The literal meaning of the word tumor is swelling or enlargement. However, on the basis of usage, the term is not applied to temporary swellings associated with acute infections, but is related instead to relatively well-defined, persistent enlargements. Tumors are classified as benign or malignant according to their manner of growth. Benign means kind or peaceful and indicates an enlarged area that tends to grow slowly in one place, and although it may displace neighboring tissues and structures, it does not invade them. Malignant means an evil thing and indicates a tumor that invades and destroys surrounding tissues and has the capacity to metasticize, that is, to migrate through the lymph or vascular systems to other sites. The tumorous nature of a disease is often designated by the suffix -oma when it is joined to a term that designates a specific type of tumor such as carcinoma, papilloma, and melanoma.

When a tumor in the larynx creates a voice change, it does so because it adds something to one or both vocal cords and thereby modifies their vibratory characteristics. It is the size and location of the tumor mass, not the type of tumor, that determines its effect on voice. However, this fact does not mean that persons concerned with voice problems are relieved of the need for familiarity with the common types of tumor; some of these neoplasms have significance beyond their immediate influence on voice.

Polyp

One form of tumor found frequently in the larynx and nose is a polyp. This term is a general label that designates an enlargement that grows from the normal surface in contrast to a tumor that develops within a structure. A polyp may be pedunculated, that is, be attached by a peduncle or stock, or it may be sessile, possessed of a broad base. The word polyp does not indicate anything about the content or character of the tumor beyond its shape and surface location. However, some physicians use the term as a clinical designation of a benign tumor.

Differentiation among polyps is designated by the type of membrane or tissue from which it arises and from the manner of its formation. Ballenger and Ballenger state that "polyps may be edematous, fibrous, cystic, or a combination of these types. For example, there are adenomatous polyps that consist of tissue derived from their glandular base; vascular polyps that are bulging angiomas (dilated lymph spaces or blood vessels); cysts that are sacs formed by blockages of ducts and may contain fluid, gas or soft material; vocal nodules that are variously designated as angioma, amyloid tumors, fibroma and localized accumulations of stratified squamous epithelium, all of which result from trauma at the site" (6). Polyps on the vocal folds may either be a localized mass or "a diffuse polypoid degeneration of both entire membranous vocal cords which has also been termed localized hypertrophic laryngitis" (8:352).

SIGNIFICANCE OF POLYPS. When polyps grow in the nose, they may reduce the space enough to impede breathing and change the resonance characteristics. Under these circumstances, if the obstruction is in the posterior part of the nasal space or in the nasopharynx, the voice will have a denasal or "cold in the head" quality. On the other hand, if the obstruction is in the anterior portion of the nasal space and if the velopharyngeal port is not closed, the nasal resonator will become a cul-de-sac and hypernasality will result. The condition can be simulated in the normal structure by pinching the nostrils and attempting to "speak through the nose."

When a localized enlargement such as a polyp is present in the larynx on either the ventricular or vocal folds, it suggests the presence of trauma, usually from vocal abuse. Unlike vocal nodules, a localized laryngeal polyp may result from a single brief period of vocal strain. If the offending structure is located on the glottal border or if it can rest on one or both vocal folds during phonation, the voice will almost always be breathy or hoarse, that is, rough-sounding. However, polyps may be located in the larynx where they do not affect vibration and be discovered only accidentally during a laryngeal examination or after complaint of discomfort. These polyps as well as those in the nose are often associated etiologically with allergies, infections, or trauma.

> 26   Luchsinger and Arnold are both physicians who have focussed much of their attention on voice disorders. Their discussion of polyps and nodules is highly instructional (58), as is the article by Arnold (1).

Vocal Nodules

Vocal nodules result from trauma to the vocal folds and develop over a period of time through several stages. They usually begin their course with edema, and if the process is not interrupted it will culminate in a well-organized, persistent fibrous polyp containing amyloid substance (starch-like) and hyalin (translucent, albuminoid substance). Nodules may also develop as a further complication of an underlying hyperplasia (see subsequent discussions of hyperplasia). These structures are usually paired and rest opposite each other on the glottal margins approximately at the midpoints of the membranous portions of the vocal folds, which is also at the junction of the anterior and middle thirds of the entire glottis. This location marks the point of widest vibratory excursion and the place of maximum pressure upon contact; consequently, it is the area of greatest trauma.

The presence of edema, which means excessive fluid in an organ or tissue, signals trauma or irritation. It frequently accompanies excessive shouting at athletic contests, prolonged loud talking or singing, and similar structurally abusive vocal activities. The vocal folds become enlarged and cause vocal disorders varying from mild hoarseness to aphonia. Usually the strenuous vocal episodes are intermittent and the larynx returns to normal between the periods of abuse. However, where traumatic use of the vocal structures becomes more or less continuous, the edematous condition is unable to subside and the swelling persists, often becoming fibrous. It is probable that a swelling, whether from hyperplasia, edema, or any other cause, intensifies the traumatic effects of contact between the vocal folds and consequently accelerates the nodular development. The sequence of histologic changes that occur in the course of nodular formation has been traced by Ash, who says there is a "beginning as a focal increase in fibrous tissue producing small swelling. In the course of time, which varies considerably in individual cases, there is a marked increase in vascularity. The blood vessels dilate more and more until the lesion becomes largely thin walled, dilated blood vessels in an edematous stroma. This is the so-called varix (permanently dilated) stage. Subsequently, a fibrinoid hyaline material is deposited in the stroma, the vessel walls, and even in their lumens. This material increases in amount and eventually dominates the picture. It is this phase that is frequently mistaken for amyloid tumor. This material is not the orthodox amyloid of diffuse amyloid disease. . . . For this reason we avoid the term amyloid tumor. . . .

"The epithelium covering the laryngeal nodule retains the squamous (scale like) type of the true cord, but it becomes very much altered in thickness, sometimes greatly reduced; at other times, the epithelium may be markedly increased in thickness with more or less parakeratosis or keratosis (horny growth of skin) over the surface" (5:245–46).

Vocal nodules are often classified as functional disorders because they are so generally related to vocal abuse. However, it is also apparent that these tumor-like structures involve tissue changes that are the direct causes of the acoustic defects of the voice. Vocal misuse contributes to a number of laryngeal changes, as has been indicated in previous discussions, without much distinction between functional or organic etiologic factors. Consequently, many voice problems can be considered to be inseparably functional and organic. The dichotomy of functional-organic becomes academic when considering such problems, but this distinction is maintained because it provides a means for systematically describing many disorders.

27   How does Murphy classify the cause of vocal nodules (71)?

Papilloma

Papilloma of the larynx is another type of tumor that frequently causes voice defects. As its name implies, it contains nipple-like masses, or papilla; these are stalks of fibrous tisue of varying thickness that branch, contain blood vessels, and are covered with squamous epithelium. Sometimes they are described as "mulberry-like nodular masses that vary in color from pinkish white to red" (7:449). Common warts represent one form of papilloma. The specific cause of papillomata is not known, but they are present in children and adults and tend to recur after removal. Viral infection has been suspected as an etiologic factor, as has chronic laryngeal irritation and some unspecified hormonal agent. This latter concept is supported by the fact that papillomas often regress at puberty. These tumors sometimes become large enough to obstruct the airway and consequently may be a threat to life. In children, papillomata in the larynx remain benign, but according to Ash, if they recur repeatedly in adults, the tumor may become malignant (5).

Papillomata may occur also at other places in the respiratory tract. They are rare in the nose, but according to Ballenger and Ballenger (7:450), are fairly common in tonsillar crypts and in the faucial area. These apparently produce but few mild symptoms in the patient and would be expected only rarely to alter nasal resonance characteristics or interfere with velopharyngeal closure.

IMPLICATIONS OF PAPILLOMA FOR THE SPEECH CLINICIAN. There is little reason to believe that vocal abuse causes papilloma or that vocal reeducation will alleviate the problem. However, a child referred for chronic hoarseness is always suspect of having this condition until a laryngeal examination demonstrates otherwise. Furthermore, since the cause of papilloma is presumed to be associated with chronic laryngeal irritation in some instances, laryngologists occasionally recommend voice therapy following removal of the tumor as an aid in reducing laryngeal abuse and the possible recurrence of the papilloma.

Cancer

This term refers generally to various types of malignant tumors, but it most commonly designates carcinoma, a neoplasm that derives from epithelial tissue. Carcinomas are the malignant tumors that are associated most frequently with the larynx and other parts of the respiratory tract, but there are other cancers, such as sarcomas and melanomas, that should also be identified since these types of tumors may also be found in the airway. Each of the common terms designating forms of cancer have many subdivisions that reveal the kinds of cell structure involved and other special characteristics of the tumor. Familiarity with them enlarges the horizons of the speech pathologist and is highly desirable for clinicians working with persons who have been treated successfully. However, the critical factors to remember about active cancer are that it is invasive, it metasticizes, and it causes death when not treated.

One of the early signs of laryngeal cancer, as is true of any other disease that interferes with vibration of the vocal cords, is a phonatory defect, that is, some form of hoarseness (20). It is rare that an individual with a persistent hoarseness seeks the advice of a speech pathologist before that of a laryngologist, but where this happens, the need for a medical evaluation before attempting voice therapy is obvious. There is no voice therapy for cancer, but there is assistance for the person who has a voice disorder as a sequel to medical therapy for the disease.

IMPLICATIONS OF LARYNGEAL CANCER. The person who has successfully faced and survived the problem of cancer in the larynx or upper respiratory tract usually has an altered speaking mechanism. He frequently also has a deep and lasting fear of a recurrence of the disease. These two factors will influence both the therapeutic procedures and the approach to the patient. The changes in the structures may vary from a minimum alteration in the laryngeal mucosa or slight atrophy of one vocal fold resulting from irradiation, to the surgical removal of part or all of the larynx. The attitudes of patients about their conditions will also vary considerably. Some are ready to look ahead to whatever rehabilitation is necessary, others remain depressed and are unwilling to respond. In the latter situations, environmental and family factors may be of great importance. It is fortunate that most patients accept whatever change has occurred and express an eagerness to cooperate in therapy.

28   There is a wealth of information in the literature about adjustment problems of the laryngectomized. The student with an interest in this

subject might start his reading with Gardner's article (*36*). Additional
material may be found in several parts of the books by Snidecor (*83*)
and Diedrich and Youngstrom (*25*). Local cancer societies often publish
pamphlets for distribution directly to patients or indirectly through
"Lost Cord" clubs. However, perhaps the most revealing account of
the problems created by cancer of the larynx is in the book by William
Gargan (*37*).

Destruction of a laryngeal carcinoma by irradiation may leave no
vocal abnormality, particularly if the lesion was treated when it was
small. In contrast, successful treatment may require extensive radiation therapy that often causes generalized changes in the laryngeal
mucosa and underlying structures. The mucous membranes may
lose their usual lubrication and the deep tissues often become fi-
brotic, less pliable, and reduced in size. These changes can alter
adduction-abduction as well as vibration and thereby influence the
severity of vocal disorders. These problems range from mild to
marked degrees of breathiness, roughness, and even to aphonia.

When surgical intervention is necessary, extensive changes in the
larynx and voice usually occur (*23*). These problems are reviewed
below in the section dealing with surgical modifications.

Hyperplasia

Hyperplasia means literally an over-formation and indicates "an
increase in the number of individual tissue elements excluding
tumor formation, whereby the bulk of the part or organ is increased" (*84*). Hyperplastic laryngitis is a chronic condition that is
marked either by localized or diffuse enlargement of the mucous
membrane and may have a seriously deleterious effect upon the
voice. It is secondary to acute attacks of laryngitis, to vocal abuse,
or to dietary deficiencies, but its specific cause is unknown. The
Ballengers state, "Hyperplastic laryngitis frequently occurs in singers due to incorrect methods of voice training and singing, using
the voice during or after colds, or from repeated attacks of throat
inflammations, both infectious and allergic" (*7*:368). It can be
observed that speakers as well as singers are subject to this condition, and it is not uncommon to observe laryngeal changes of this
type in children who use their voices excessively.

The localized form of hyperplasia may appear in various sites
within the larynx. It is often displayed as swelling on the vocal folds
that extends from the anterior commissure posteriorly along part or

all of the membranous glottis. The condition may also be observed as swollen, rounded ridges parallel to the glottal border in the subglottal area or as a circumscribed enlargement of the mucous membrane in the posterior commissure. It is noted that edema is an intimate and significant factor that is regularly associated with these displays of localized hyperplasia in the larynx.

Swelling along the anterior segments of the vocal folds from hyperplasia, edema, or other causes, seriously impairs their vibration. Such enlargements even when small are often squeezed between the anterior borders of the glottis, thereby effectively limiting the length of the membranous folds and causing a higher pitch. More extensive anterior swelling may raise the pitch in a similar manner, and also create some form of hoarseness by causing irregular vibration, produce breathiness by preventing glottal closure, or cause aphonia by interfering completely with vibration. It is probable that hyperplasia localized in the immediate area of the anterior commissure frequently escapes detection, since it can be seen clearly only when the commissure is visible and the folds are abducted. If the subglottal swellings that are sometimes described as being sausage-like are large enough to intrude into the glottal area, they may vibrate during phonation. When this occurs, a low pitched vocal sound is produced that may have a prominent roughness associated with it. Localized enlargement in the posterior glottis may interfere with adduction and thereby affect voice, but this change will not occur unless the swelling is unusually large. Swelling that is limited to the posterior regions usually does not involve the membranous glottis and consequently exerts little influence upon vibration.

Persons with chronic hoarseness and no recognized specific laryngeal disturbance to account for the voice disorder may have a generalized hyperplasia of the vocal folds. A slight, more or less uniform enlargement may not be identified readily, particularly if the larynx is not inflamed and if the structure had not been observed prior to the vocal disturbance. Since hyperplasia increases the mass and probably the compliance of the vibrators, the pitch of the voice is predictably lower and it may be rough sounding. However, as indicated in the earlier discussion, when there is an additional fullness in the folds at the anterior commissure, the vibrators may be partially damped and their frequency raised.

IMPLICATIONS OF HYPERPLASIA. One implication of the preceding discussion is that a relatively subtle change in the vocal cords may cause any of several possible vocal disturbances. The variability of vocal symptoms supports the contention that the nature of laryngeal disease cannot be determined by the vocal sound produced. However, awareness of the kinds of vibratory changes that are associated with certain vocal characteristics or modifications enables the speech pathologist, and others sensitive to the sound produced, to recognize the nature of the organic deviations that are present.

Another implication is that both general and localized hyperplasia of the vocal cords may cause phonatory problems more frequently than has been generally recognized. The need for careful and detailed evaluation of the various possible associated etiologic factors becomes evident in each individual case.

Keratosis

Keratosis denotes an area on the epidermis that has an outgrowth of the horny layer. Keratin is the name for the material of which horn and the outer layer of the skin is composed. The disease causes the mucosa to become thickened, stiffened, and irregular, particularly along the glottal borders. Keratosis often accompanies hyperplasia and may cause irregular, hard, white areas on the vocal folds. The exact cause of the condition is not known, but it is thought to result from a food or vitamin deficiency.

Keratosis is introduced to this discussion because hoarseness is its primary symptom. Its treatment initially is medical; subsequently, if vocal abuse were related to the accompanying hyperplasia, vocal reeducation might be indicated.

*Additional Localized Factors that Influence
Vocal Cord Vibration*

It was pointed out variously in the preceding paragraphs that tumors and tumor-like lesions ordinarily alter the mass, shape, and movements of laryngeal structures or reduce the size of the respiratory space and thereby detrimentally influence either vocal cord vibration or resonance. Similar effects of a localized mechanical type may also result from a variety of non-tumorous diseases and organic changes, such as laryngeal web, contact ulcer, irritating substances, fractures and other injuries, and surgery. It is important that persons interested in voice disorders also understand the nature of these other disturbances and recognize their significance.

Laryngeal Web

A laryngeal web is a membranous partition that extends across the glottis from one vocal fold to another. It is usually located in the anterior part of the larynx and varies in size from a small membrane filling the anterior commissure to a structure that extends to the vocal processes of the arytenoid cartilages, thereby occluding most of the airway. Webs may also be found connecting the ventricular folds or spanning the larynx subglottally. These structures are either congenital, the cause of which is unknown, or cicatricial, resulting from injury or surgery at the contacting parts of the vocal folds.

29   Follow this brief sketch on laryngeal web with the article by Poe and Seager (76).

SIGNIFICANCE OF WEBS. If a laryngeal web is extensive, it interferes with breathing, causing both respiratory difficulty and stridor. Usually these conditions are readily observed even in an infant, and appropriate medical attention can be provided. Conversely, when a web is relatively small, its presence may not be detected until such time as its effect on the voice causes it to be discovered.

A web shortens the free margins of the vocal folds and prevents air flow at its location, thereby changing the potential vibratory characteristics of the system. The web membrane probably folds and contracts into a wedge of tissue that is compressed into the anterior commissural area during adduction for phonation. The tissue mass restricts the freedom of the vocal folds anteriorly and effectively shortens their vibrating portions. This modification probably accounts for the high pitch that characteristically accompanies the smaller laryngeal webs. The slight hoarseness that is also present frequently results undoubtedly from vibratory irregularity and glottal air leak that are caused by the web.

Contact Ulcer

In 1928, C. L. Jackson described a condition that he named "contact ulcer," which is characterized by an ulcer or ulcers located on the opposing surfaces of one or both arytenoid cartilages (45). The lesions occur on the medial aspects of the vocal processes where the cartilages come in contact with each other in a manner referred to by Jackson as "a hammer and anvil." The ulcers are shallow, being formed in the relatively thin mucosal covering of the cartilage, and they frequently support granulation tissue. These ulcers occasionally cause localized pain in the larynx and sometimes produce sharp pain referred to the ear on the involved side. Slight hoarseness is a frequent symptom and may be the first evidence of the underlying lesion.

Vocal abuse composed of frequent effortful speaking at low pitch seems to contribute to contact ulcer formation (8:332–33). It is also probable that there are additional contributing etiologic factors, such as infections in the tonsils or elsewhere, irritating dusts or smoke, coughing, and other behavioral trauma. A unilateral contact ulcer is known to have developed following a single two minute period of low pitched, grunting phonation that was associated with repetitive vigorous contact between the arytenoid cartilages (89). It is probable that the formation and persistence of contact ulcers is facilitated by the rubbing of the arytenoid cartilages upon each other as they are vibrated by vocal cord action at low pitch.

IMPLICATIONS OF CONTACT ULCER. The presence of a contact ulcer signals vocal abuse and indicates that the underlying condition will not be alleviated successfully until the use of the voice has been modified. The hoarseness is caused primarily by swelling of the laryngeal mucosa that results from engorgement of the minute blood vessels in areas of the vocal cords adjacent to the ulcer. The general absence of pain and only occasional consciousness of laryngeal discomfort accompanied by relatively mild hoarseness support the belief that many patients who request vocal assistance have had their contact ulcers for considerable periods of time. The relative prevalence of the condition among men and the characteristic effortful low pitch suggest the possible importance of occupation, environment, and personality as etiologic factors.

Contact ulcer is not typically considered to be precancerous, but malignant lesions have developed in regions previously occupied by contact ulcer. Consequently, it is important that a person who has the condition remain under the surveillance of a laryngologist during vocal therapy (9).

Irritating Substances

There are several kinds of irritants that can cause inflammation of the mucosal surfaces of both the larynx and nose and which, consequently, may alter the voice. Some of these substances are carried in the air; others may be applied directly to the surfaces. The former include dusts, pollens, and powdered materials of various kinds that may be mechanically irritating, chemically irritating, or may cause an allergic response. Other airborne irritants, such as vapors, fumes, gases and smoke from various burning substances, including tobacco, also cause changes in the mucosa and sometimes the underlying structures. In some instances, even prolonged exposure to extremely dry air can damage the mucous membranes and thereby contribute to both phonatory and resonance disorders. It is stressed in the literature that the impairment of the larynx from all these substances is greater in mouth breathers.

The irritants that are applied directly to the membranes come from improper or excessive application of medicaments, swallowing of caustic and similar substances, or flow of material from infected areas in adjacent parts of the respiratory tract. The irritating substances of a chemical nature that are swallowed rarely affect the interior of the larynx directly. However, inflammation in the pharynx can result in excessive mucus and edema in the vocal fold area.

Inflammations of the nasal or laryngeal mucosa exert their deleterious effects on the voice, primarily through the swelling or drying of the surface membranes or combinations of these factors. Dilation of the minute blood vessels, associated with related edema, causes an engorgement of the mucosa that reduces the size of the resonator and modifies both the compliance and mass of the vocal folds. These changes tend to lower vocal pitch and alter nasal resonance, as when a head cold is present. Conversely, drying of the surfaces tends to increase the viscosity of the mucus and to cause crusting in both the nose and larynx. These conditions create discomfort, coughing, and impairment of vibration. The changes in vocal fold motion accompanying the drying and other mucosal deterioration have not been studied in detail, but it is probable that the organic modifications contribute transient elements to the vibratory pattern and also reduce the pliability of the folds. Such variations would be expected to produce a relatively weak voice, lacking in vitality and containing high frequency noise elements.

SIGNIFICANCE OF IRRITANTS. When a fireman, for example, accidentally inhales damaging amounts of smoke or fumes, this fact is recognized immediately and the influence on both structure and voice can be readily and directly assessed. Fortunately, such accidents occur infrequently and rarely involve rehabilitation. However, considerable impairment to the respiratory and vocal mechanisms of persons in the general population probably occurs from inconspicuous inflammatory substances that exist in occupational or home environments and which exert their influences cumulatively over considerable periods of time. This possibility demonstrates that the speech clinician needs to investigate these potentially irritating factors along with the pattern of vocal use, particularly when the amount and kind of speaking or singing does not support a diagnosis limited to vocal abuse. With suitable mucosal conditions, a mild amount of vocal misuse could cause excessive vocal deviation. The presence of inflammation and associated edema in the vocal folds provides an ideal basis for vocal deterioration. When the history and vocal condition do not indicate strongly that vocal abuse was etiologically significant, vocal reeducation should be limited or postponed until the environmental and health factors have been carefully assessed.

> 30   The irritants previously discussed often produce a chronic laryngitis. The presentation by DeWeese and Saunders (24:134–35) provides much insight on this subject.

Fractures and Other Injuries

Localized changes in the larynx or nose resulting from fractures or dislocations may cause vocal disorders. When the larynx is injured in an automobile accident or by some other violent traumatic event, there may be a fracture of one or more of the laryngeal cartilages or dislocations at the cricothyroid or cricoarytenoid articulations. Following the maximum possible surgical restoration, structural deviations, such as asymmetries of the two sides, shortening of the vocal folds, partial collapse of the internal laryngeal structures, or limitation of motion of the arytenoid or thyroid cartilages, may remain. The laryngeal changes can cause abnormal vocal pitch or hoarseness of many kinds.

Fractures of the nose affect the voice when they result in reduction in size or stoppage of the airway. The septum and other structures inside the nose may be displaced laterally or depressed to produce firm obstructions. However, some of these injuries may not in themselves stop the flow of sound and air, but they can create conditions that allow the accumulation of mucus that effectively blocks the passage.

IMPLICATIONS OF FRACTURES AND OTHER INJURIES. Vocal disorders resulting from fractures of the nose or larynx and dislocation in the latter are rare. However, when the trauma affects the larynx, the implications for the speech clinician are extensive. He should realize that the condition may be a threat to life through suffocation and consequently that therapy must be instituted only when it is advised by the patient's physician. Vocal therapy may be useful as part of the general rehabilitation process as well as an aid in the restoration of phonation, but it should always be conducted in close collaboration with the otolaryngologist, at least until the post-traumatic condition is stabilized. The speech clinician should remember that any serious accident involving the head or neck may have produced multiple injuries affecting the thyroid gland, spinal column, brain and spinal cord, peripheral nerves, or blood supply. Therapy without recognition of such potentials may result in unsatisfactory progress and frustrations for everyone involved.

31 The tragic increase of throat injury in automobile accidents makes it mandatory to read the article by Butler and Moser (16).

Surgical Alteration of the Larynx

The paralyses, tumors of various kinds, and the other laryngeal conditions that were reviewed earlier in this chapter are associated closely with the present consideration of surgical intervention. The previous discussions touched upon conditions that may require surgery. It seems appropriate here to recognize briefly those changes that may persist subsequent to operative procedures and which form the bases for voice disorders.

Surgical intervention in the larynx usually implies the removal of tissue and may be classified according to the extensiveness of the surgical modifications and their effects upon phonation. The first and simplest of these procedures includes the removal of polyps or other masses from the surface without involvement of underlying tissue; usually there are no subsequent detrimental effects on the voice. The second type of intervention is related to the maintenance of an adequate airway in such conditions as bilateral paralysis or comparable obstructive conditions. The procedures include the lateral fixation of one vocal fold, the removal of an arytenoid cartilage, and the lateral placement of the remaining structures or the excision of hyperplastic or other tissue. Since glottal closure usually cannot be achieved following such changes, the vocal sound tends to be breathy and weak. The voice may also be hoarse as a consequence of irregular vibratory movements of the involved structures, particularly when a loud sound is attempted. The third degree of involvement includes extensive excision of intrinsic laryngeal tissue, usually most or all of one vocal fold. When a tumor or other condition invades the deep structures of a fold, that member usually is removed, thereby creating a permanently open glottis and an inefficient vibrator. The resulting voice can be aphonic, but it is more likely to be weak, breathy, and hoarse. The latter feature results from the vibrations of vicarious structures, such as the ventricular cords, epiglottis, or mucosal folds that are brought into proximity with the healthy vocal cord or other structures on the opposite side of the larynx. The fourth and most extensive surgical procedure involving the larynx is its total removal. When this occurs, the upper respiratory tract is altered extensively, the individual is forced to breath through a stoma in his neck, and he is unable to produce sound in an ordinary manner. Such persons may learn to substitute a vicarious natural sound source, such as the upper part of the esophagus, that can produce a controlled, modified eructation; or they may use an artificial electrical or mechanical sound source that introduces sound into the upper respiratory area. The larynx normally produces a phonetically undifferentiated sound that is molded into meaningful utterance by the movements of the oral structures. Any other complex sound that is put into the mouth and pharynx can also be modified into language by the customary articulatory adjustments.

SIGNIFICANCE OF SURGICAL ALTERATIONS. Surgical modification of the larynx that results in a vocal disorder reflects the fact that the remaining structure is abnormal, that the patient may be emotionally upset, particularly if a cancer has been present, and that vocal reeducation will require the learning of compensatory phonatory adjustments. Often the voice will remain permanently abnormal, but training frequently enables the person to produce adequately loud, intelligible speech with relatively little effort. An understanding of laryngeal mechanics and the organic modifications that have been produced in a specific patient are essentials in therapy.

32   To gain an understanding of the physical and physiological conditions present in laryngectomized persons, see the report by Robe and others (78) and also several appropriate sections in the books by Diedrich and Youngstrom (25) and Snidecor (83).

LARYNGEAL IMPAIRMENTS CAUSED BY SYSTEMIC CONDITIONS AND NON-LOCALIZED DISEASES

In the preceding section, the emphasis was on the organic disorders that are localized in the larynx without close association with generalized diseases or physical conditions. The following discussion focuses on diseases and conditions that are less specific to the larynx but which involve the vocal folds and consequently the voice. The two primary mechanisms through which the generalized conditions influence the larynx are edema and fatigue. A few incidental references to edema have already been made, but it is essential that the speech pathologist have a relatively complete understanding of edema and its causes. It is also desirable to have some insight into hormonal influences, anemia, and the mechanisms of fatigue.

Edema and Its Significance in Voice Disorders

Edema, which means a swelling resulting from the presence of serous fluid in extra vascular spaces, has been mentioned previously in association with inflammation, trauma, and various diseases. It is probably apparent that edema is not a disease; it is a condition that causes localized or generalized enlargement of a structure or area. When it is present in the vocal cords, it affects their mass, elasticity, and compliance, with a consequent influence on phonation. Edema may follow weakening of the walls of the capillary vessels by local injury; it may be associated with inflammatory diseases; it may also result from obstruction of the veins or lymph channels; and it may be caused by certain medicaments, glandular imbalance, and allergenic substances. Non-inflammatory edema is as vocally detrimental as edema from other causes, and it is probably more common. Edema in its minor degrees is difficult to recognize, but in certain locations in the larynx, particularly at or near the anterior commissure, even minor swelling may have vocally detrimental effects similar to those associated with hyperplasia in that area.

Obstructions affecting the flow of venous blood or lymph can be caused by mechanical compression from such factors as constriction of venal channels, a growth pressing on a vein, or any condition that reduces the flow and causes an increase in pressure on the supply side of the obstruction. This condition causes the serous fluid to move through the minute blood vessel walls into the surrounding areas or impedes the flow of lymph in its channels.

The internal medicaments that may cause edema include the iodides and acetylsalicylic acid (aspirin). The iodides, particularly potassium iodide and sodium iodide, which are used in the treatment of bronchial and certain other respiratory diseases, liquify and accelerate secretions of the mucosa and tend to produce edema in the process. Jackson and Jackson state that the selective effect of potassium iodide on the larynx "may go so far as to produce acute edema of the larynx or a chronic engorgement" (46:55).

Glandular imbalance, particularly hypothyroidism, produces its detrimental vocal effects through edema. The disturbance need not be great to influence the voice, and since persons with borderline hypothyroid conditions frequently are not aware of their disorders, it is probable that many of the mild, so-called functional cases of hoarseness are caused by thyroid imbalance (59). Variations in gonadal function also influence fluid balance and consequently affect the voice. The most frequent evidence of this condition is the change of voice noticed by many women in relation to their menstrual cycles (34). Usually, the vocal problem lasts for only a few days, but in some women it is persistent.

Allergic reactions take many forms but often appear as either localized or generalized edematous swellings; that is, edema is frequently the evidence of a reaction to an allergin. The respiratory tract may be the site of this reaction and the larynx is usually involved. The implication of these two factors is that the reaction may affect breathing as well as the larynx and thereby further complicate the voice problem.

Allergy is an exaggerated sensitivity to substances or situations. The changes that occur can be brought on by pollens, foods, drugs, molds, physical agents such as cold and barometric changes, and emotional disturbances.

"A large number of theories have been advanced to explain the allergic reaction, but no simple one has been found satisfactory to account for all the observed phenomena. It seems likely that a great variety of things happen as a result of the introduction of an allergen into a sensitive person. One of these is the liberation of histamine, a powerful substance that causes smooth muscle contractions, capillary dilatation and fall in blood pressure. Other substances liberated probably include acetylcholine, heparin, and serotonin. It is probable that many more such substances are liberated by the cells of the body when they are injured. The mechanism by which the cells are injured is equally obscure. It is generally believed, however, that the basis of allergy is a reaction between the allergen and a body protein called an antibody" (29).

The multiple causes of edema and its effect on the voice when the larynx is involved stress the potential importance of this condition in the evaluation and management of voice disorders. Extra vascular fluid, whether it be caused by disease, trauma, interference with fluid distribution, medicaments, glandular imbalance or allergic reactions, modifies the behavior of the vocal cords and consequently the vocal sound. Its subtle presence serves to obscure diagnosis and complicate therapy. Its potential importance to the voice pathologist cannot be over emphasized.

Hormonal Influence

In the preceding section on edema, endocrine imbalance was included as one cause. Endocrine disturbances may also influence voice by disturbing the growth of the vocal folds. In the male, the failure of gonadal development before puberty retards laryngeal development and results in a female-type larynx and voice. In the adult female, virilization (masculinization) of the voice sometimes follows the medical administration of anabolic steroids (18 and *19*). The precise mechanism by which the change in the vocal folds occurs is not known at this time, but since the condition is irreversible, it is presumed that the vibrating structures become more massive through a hyperplastic process.

IMPLICATIONS OF HORMONAL INFLUENCES ON VOICE. Modern medical therapy is able to compensate to a considerable degree for the failure of gonadal development in the young boy. Consequently, it is unlikely that the speech pathologist will be called upon for therapy unless habit patterns cause the juvenile voice to persist after medically induced laryngeal development has occurred.

At the present time, the laryngeal changes causing virilization of the female voice are permanent. Women having this distressing condition can be helped somewhat through the emphasis of female speech patterns and the raising of the vocal pitch, but the general prognosis is not favorable.

Anemia

Anemia, which means an inadequate blood supply to a muscle, organ, membrane or other structure, presents among its symptoms muscular weakness and paleness of the mucosa and skin. The deficiency in the blood may be in its content, that is, a "dimunition of the amount of hemoglobin . . . or of the number of red corpuscles or both . . . or the condition may result from local reduction in the blood supply, or by compression of a vessel, embolism, spasm, etc.; . . ." (*27*). It should be apparent to the speech pathologist that anemia is an expression of a variety of underlying conditions, including nutrition and disease.

SIGNIFICANCE OF ANEMIA IN VOCAL DISORDERS. When chronic muscular weakness or quick fatigability are present in the larynx or the muscles of respiration, the voice is usually weak and breathy. It deteriorates with prolonged speaking and improves following rest. Individuals rarely express primary concern for their voices when anemia is present in a marked degree; at that time they seek medical treatment. However, they may inquire of the speech pathologist about a change or inadequacy of voice when a mild anemia is present. Usually such patients are not aware of their physical condition, or if they are, they do not associate the blood deficiency with their vocal symptoms. Muscular fatigue may contribute directly to vocal weakness and breathy quality through its effect on respiratory control and regulation of the glottis. It may also act indirectly to cause compensatory over-reactions of adductor muscles, which results in inefficient or detrimental phonatory behavior. These latter deviations may produce tremulousness, vocal roughness, and glottalization or vocal fry.

RETROSPECT

A number of pathologies that can affect voice have been presented briefly in this chapter for five purposes: (1) to provide the speech pathologist and clinician with basic information about organic deviations that are frequently unfamiliar to him; (2) to encourage him to search further into these and other pertinent organic etiologic factors; (3) to foster an alertness to and an awareness of the possible significance of abnormalities or changes in size, color, motion, and behavior of the structures used in voice production; (4) to provide certain insights that may be useful in diagnosis of voice disorders; and (5) to stress by inference and indirection that remediation for voice disorders usually encompasses more than an assessment of the voice and a set of vocal exercises.

DIAGNOSIS IS THE PROCESS OF DISCOVERING THE CAUSE OF CERTAIN symptoms. Diagnosis of voice disorders ordinarily encompasses the recognition and description of individual vocal deviations and a systematic search for the factors that cause these deviations.

The critical word in the preceding statement is "cause." This concept seems simple, but when the diagnostic procedures reveal, for example, that a specific vocal disorder is "caused" by vocal nodules, are the nodules really the "cause"? Undoubtedly, the audible symptoms result from the presence of nodules, but it has been established that nodules are themselves symptoms of other causes. Since one of the long-standing axioms of therapy is that treatment must be focused on causes, not on symptoms, which of the several causes should be treated? It should be apparent that the ultimate or pri-

5 *diagnostic procedures*

mary cause, in whatever hierarchy of causes may exist, ideally should receive the major therapeutic attention. Yet, the primary cause may not be amenable to therapy, or it may no longer exist. It is often apparent that remedial attention to one or more of the secondary causes is the only rational therapeutic approach. Diagnosis is probably the most important single aspect of a remedial program. It is based on knowledge and experience; it determines the direction and sets the pattern for everything that follows. The need for thorough preparation and alert observations cannot be stressed too strongly. Diagnosis begins when an individual, a person who is unlike any other person, presents himself to you, the diagnostician, because his voice does not sound the way he or someone else believes it should. It is from this moment in the first meeting that the clinician employs his knowledge and skill to identify, to describe, and to discover the causes of a specific voice disorder. To know theory, to know in general about diagnosis and therapy for voice defects is sterile information until it is shaped to an individual.

Several books have been published in speech pathology and
108 audiology that provide detailed guides to successful diagnosis (*21*

and 52). The following presentation does not presume to replace or to better them; it is included for purposes of emphasis. The student should develop his diagnostic methods from a combination of sources, including his own unique background and insights. Perfection in diagnosis can be approached, but it is an art that lends itself continuously to study, practice, and improvement, without much chance of achieving the ultimate.

33   The "guiding principles" of diagnosis and appraisal set forth by Darley (21:1–14) are absolutely essential for all persons working in speech pathology. The remainder of that book should be used as a companion for the suggestions presented here.

THE PATIENT'S VIEWPOINT

The sensitive diagnostician recognizes that an individual arrives for his initial meeting after certain events have occurred and concepts have been developed. An appointment has been made at a particular place and possibly with a specified clinician. The applicant may have received a questionnaire in the mail asking for much information that is more or less closely associated in his thinking with his voice disorder. He may have been asked also to see an otolaryngologist. The person who has the voice problem that has precipitated the appointment may be eager for the meeting, but, in contrast, he may be fearful or apprehensive. His attitudes will be influenced by a great variety of factors, including his age, the source of his referral, his family, his occupation, and his concept of his voice. The child with a faulty voice who is "discovered" by a speech clinician in a school survey or by the classroom teacher is usually unconcerned about his voice. His mother may share his attitude, or she may be either genuinely worried about the problem or antagonistic about the whole idea. The adult who has been referred for voice therapy by a physician may comprehend the nature of his problem and approach therapy eagerly and with confidence. On the other hand, he may question his doctor's judgment and be apprehensive about cancer or other serious disease, particularly if there has been a history of malignancy or respiratory disorders in his family. He may be upset by other members of his immediate family who have expressed their concerns. It should be noted that these worries are related primarily to the possible implications of the voice disorder, not the disorder itself. In contrast, the singer, preacher, or actor, whose voice is vital in his professional work, is concerned about the sound of the voice itself as well as the reasons for its failure and the remedial steps necessary for restoration. His level of anxiety may be high, not so much because he fears disease but because he visualizes loss of his position and income. The experienced clinician recognizes the existence of these many possible attitudes and is alert to their potential influence from the first moment of the initial meeting.

THE CLINICAL SETTING

Other factors in the environment that can influence the success of the initial diagnostic session include the conduct of the professional staff and the appearance of the physical facility. The offices and rooms to which the patient (or client) comes, whether they are in a school or a speech and hearing center, need not be elaborate or large, but they should be clean and neat. Unattractive, cluttered space tends to destroy the patient's confidence in the qualifications of the professional personnel. In contrast, favorable attitudes are engendered when each staff member is friendly, focuses his attention completely on the individual, and approaches him with appropriate dignity and respect. It is also essential that the responsible professional person remain in complete charge of the situation; that he be able and willing to take the lead and direct the interview, examination, or test. He should not exhibit any sense of hurry, but he must remember that he has no time to waste.

The diagnostic staff ideally should consist of several speech pathologists, an audiologist, an otolaryngologist, a clinical psychologist, and a social worker. Unfortunately, this array of personnel is usually not available; the speech pathologist often works alone and must call on the persons in the related professions through referral. This latter situation places great professional and ethical demands upon the independent worker. He must at once be qualified to carry his evaluation far enough to determine the need for referral and yet avoid encroachment into the areas of other professions. Experience with the former clarifies the latter.

PLAN OF THE DIAGNOSTIC SESSION

The speech pathologist should establish and follow a regular plan of diagnostic procedure that progresses systematically. Varying amounts of preliminary historical information and different vocal symptoms will modify the evaluative items in each case, but by the end of the diagnostic session the speech pathologist should have obtained and compiled the following eight kinds of information: (1) a description of the patient's voice (and any other existing speech problems); (2) a history of the disorder and of those events in the individual's life that appear to be related to the problem; (3) a description of the speech mechanism and its characteristic behavior; (4) an audiometric evaluation commensurate with indicated needs; (5) a determination of the need for referral for additional information; (6) a summary of findings through staff discussion; (7) a diagnosis or tentative diagnosis; and (8) recommendations written and discussed with the patient when such discussion is appropriate. The kinds of information needed determine the steps in the diagnostic session, but the sequence listed above, particularly the first four units, need not be developed in any particular order. The unique elements in each patient-diagnostician meeting require flexibility and variation. However, a possible sequence of procedures is presented in the following discussion by tracing a progression of evaluative steps from the initial patient-clinician meeting until the end of the session.

INITIAL PHASE OF THE DIAGNOSTIC PROCESS. Diagnosis begins when the patient arrives. Evaluation of his voice starts with the first exchange of greetings and continues throughout the period of the meeting. Similarly, assessments of coordination and locomotor skill are derived from unobstrusive observations of walking, sitting, standing, motions of the arms, and facial expressions. Appraisal of these movements and adjustments will occur throughout the diagnostic procedure, but one of the best opportunities to attend to them is at the time the interviewer shakes hands with the patient and ushers him into the office or room where the case history will be taken. Unusual, even subtle abnormalities, may reflect neural disorders or past injuries and diseases that have influenced voice or speech. Exploratory questions of the types indicated below ordinarily establish the importance of the observed symptoms in relation to the voice or speech problem.

When the patient, or a parent with his child, is conducted to the conference room or area, he should be directed to a chair and invited to sit down. This chair should be located on the opposite side of the desk from the interviewer and far enough away to prevent the patient from reading the notes that will be written. If the patient is a child, he should be seated close to his parent for optimum management purposes. Questioning begins with those items of identification that are not already available from referral information or that should be reviewed for confirmation. Where possible, the child should be encouraged to reply to questions to enable the interviewer to hear his voice and speech. If the patient is an adult, the replies that he gives in this routine questioning will reveal enough of the nature of his voice to indicate that the primary deviation is a resonance problem, a phonatory disorder, or a combination of such differences. Within this brief period the interviewer will have noted the presence of any hyper- or hypo-nasality as well as gross pitch deviations, relative loudness, breathi-ness, or hoarseness. This early general evaluation frequently assists the clinician in formulating his questions more effectively through-out the remainder of the interview.

PATIENT'S ASSESSMENT OF HIS VOICE. The next logical inquiry fo-cuses upon the patient's concept of his voice. The exact wording of questions will vary with the specific circumstances, but possible approaches are "What comments have been made about your voice?" "Why did you decide to come here for assistance with your voice?" His answers may not only provide valuable diagnostic infor-mation, they also will reveal his insight and general comprehension of his vocal disorder.

The previous questions lead naturally to inquiries about the beginning of the disorder. These include questions about the date or period of time in which the problem began or was first noticed; the circumstances that the patient associates with its initiation; the course of its development; his attitude toward it and his previous attempts to modify it. Of course, if the voice problem began with a recognized specific disease, injury, or surgical procedure, the his-tory is relatively simple. It is the indefinite initiation that taxes and challenges the interviewer. Obscure recollection of the problem is characteristic in the histories of children's voices because these are subject to frequent acute variation, so that parents rarely realize when a chronic disorder has become established. Furthermore, most parents rarely remember a date or a period when a certain event occurred, unless they considered it to be particularly serious or unless it happened in relation to some other noteworthy occasion. The fact that a parent remembers something about the child's voice may indicate his recognition of the potential gravity of the problem.

If the speech pathologist who conducts the case history interview also evaluates the voice, it is often wise to interrupt the history review at this point and to shift the attention to the voice proper. This procedure enables the examiner to assess the voice in detail and to discover possible areas of importance about which questions should be asked when the history interview is resumed.

Evaluation of the Voice

The steps in voice assessment that are outlined below are useful and practical, but there should be no compulsion to follow them rigidly. The order of progression has no particular value and it is not always necessary or desirable to include all parts of the evaluation. The important need is to hear the voice as it is customarily used and to sample its potential capabilities in pitch, loudness, and quality.

Whenever possible, the voice assessment should be recorded; when the interviewing office is not too noisy, it is efficient to have the recorder immediately available, so that turning to it progresses smoothly without appreciable interruption in the interview. However, if it is necessary to go out of the office to an acoustically treated room or booth, suitable comments to the patient about the need to use good equipment or to move to a quiet area are accepted readily. Informal comments to the patient such as, "We want to have some samples of your voice as it is today for possible comparison with it at a later time." or "Part of our regular procedure is the recording of voices; have you ever recorded your voice before?" usually allay shyness or reluctance about speaking into a microphone. The person should be told that he will be asked to talk a little about a hobby or something else that interests him, to read a short paragraph, and to do a few other things.

The subject is asked to give his name, address, and the date as the recording machine is started. This step is stressed because it becomes vitally important later for identification and because even experienced clinicians occasionally forget to request it. Questions should continue immediately about a hobby, a recent vacation, interest in sports or scouting or school or occupation, and so on. If, during the preceding interview the patient spoke readily about his voice problem and its history, he should be asked to comment on it again. The recording of his narrative will be useful, not only as a voice sample but also for verification of the previous report. The extemporaneous comments of the patient should be interrupted at an appropriate point after a minute or two, and a short paragraph of relatively simple material given to him to read. If the individual is too young or for other reasons does not read, he should be urged to recite a poem, nursery rhyme, prayer, or some other material.

During this speaking and reading stage in the vocal assessment, the subject reveals his usual patterns of speaking. To analyze or to discover special features or limitations of the voice, it is desirable to focus on special vocal tasks that demonstrate discrete abilities and defects. To observe performance under respiratory stress and to note control of the breath supply, the subject can be asked to take a deep breath and count as far as possible on one breath. This counting should be repeated three times to provide an adequate sample. For variety, the alphabet can be used equally well. Prolonged speaking on one breath gives indication of the individual's competence and efficiency of phonation. However, the actual time of the utterance probably has no more validity as a measure of laryngeal efficiency than the prolongation of vowel sounds (77).

If the average pitch level has been within normal limits, the second analytical step is to survey the individual's capacity to recognize and to regulate his pitch. Ask the patient to hum a sound at a middle or comfortable pitch and to go up a scale by steps as far as possible. Since many persons have trouble recognizing pitch and producing a scale, it is often necessary for the examiner to present a sample tone to start the subject, and it may also be necessary to intone each note in the scale as a stimulus for the patient. After going up the scale, the initial middle pitch should be sounded again and the subject helped to go down the scale as far as possible. Immediately, the humming tone should be replaced by an "oh" or "ah" sound and the upward and downward scale range repeated. These scale maneuvers reveal the pitch range of the patient and his ability to match and to control his pitch, the degree of openness of the nasal passages as demonstrated by the humming, and changes in the excellence or defectiveness of phonation that may become apparent in different regions of the scale. These vocal performances indicate the possibility of organic disorders that can be investigated in the subsequent examination of the vocal mechanism.

> 34   One of the most concrete guides for evaluation of voice disorders is presented by Van Riper (87:467–71).

The third step in the analysis of the voice probes the individual's ability to change the loudness of his voice. Explain the purpose, and ask the patient to speak a little louder into the microphone as he counts from 1 to 5. Follow with instructions to repeat with a louder voice and then still louder until he demonstrates a very loud voice or what appears to be his maximum effort. If the loud voice causes pain or discomfort, the test should be terminated and the structure explored subsequently to discover the source of the physical discomfort. It is presumed that the examiner will adjust the recorder to compensate for the louder voice to avoid distortion of the recording.

Some persons, particularly children and women, find it difficult to speak loudly in a small room. This problem can be overcome frequently by introducing a loud noise through earphones and, while the noise is present, asking the individual to count as suggested previously.

Attempts to speak loudly demonstrate the patient's capacity to control his voice; they sometimes reveal his breathing habits under effortful conditions; and they may change the quality of his voice. Deviations in these items require attention in the subsequent examination of the mechanism, and they may be directly relevant in therapy.

A fourth analytical step searches for variations in the voice disorder associated with different vowel sounds. Occasionally a voice will sound less defective, or perhaps more defective, when certain vowels are produced. To perform this part in the assessment the examiner should ask the subject to repeat after him a series of vowel sounds that can be prolonged, and each should be initiated with [h]; e.g. hi, heɪ, hæ, hɑ, hɔ, hou, hu, hʌ, hɝ, haɪ, hau, hɔɪ. The results may be useful in subsequent therapy.

> 35   The presence of nasalization or denasalization can be detected readily in spontaneous speech, reading, and the production of isolated syllables that do not contain nasal sounds. However, special procedures are

often needed to determine the degree of nasality in children. How
applicable are the procedures suggested by McWilliams and Musgrave (61)?

At the completion of the vocal evaluation it may be desirable or
necessary to resume the history interview, but where that can be
postponed until after the organs of speech have been examined, it
is helpful to do so. Conditions are frequently observed during the
examination that need to be pursued by further questioning.

Observation of the Speech Mechanism

Speech pathologists necessarily build therapy for voice disorders
in conformity with the vocal needs of each individual afflicted. It is
essential that all relevant material on each patient and his voice
be obtained, including an analysis of the condition and behavior of
the organs that produce voice. To obtain such knowledge this
mechanism of speech must be observed, and the speech pathologist
should be capable of accomplishing that task; it is part of his
responsibility. As indicated earlier, it would be desirable to have
an otolaryngologist on the diagnostic staff for immediate assessment
of health and medical problems associated with voice defects, but
whether the medical report is received before, during, or after the
diagnostic session, the speech pathologist still needs to conduct his
own unique type of evaluation. It is a rare otolaryngologist who
professes to know much about the functioning of the several parts
of the respiratory tract as a coordinated phonatory mechanism.

For many years experimental phoneticians and speech clinicians
have routinely observed the movements associated with breathing
and adjustments of tongue and velum during voice production.
A few have also observed the interior of the larynx with a mirror,
but some have been unwilling to develop this simple skill. Such
reluctance is unfortunate and represents a failure of responsibility
among speech pathologists. One reason expressed for this attitude
is the fear that such activity would encroach on the practice of
medicine. The opinion expressed here is that looking at the interior
of the larynx during the production of voice does not involve the
practice of medicine any more than observing the adjustment of
the lips in the production of plosive sounds. The fact that some
of the techniques employed in viewing the larynx may be shared by

physicians, speech pathologists, and phoneticians does not imply medical practice.

It is presumed, of course, that the examiner has learned how to conduct the examination and that he has practiced it sufficiently to enable him to perform it deftly. It is also presumed that the speech pathologist is completely familiar with the appearance and various behaviors of the structures he is observing. Anything less would constitute unethical practice in speech pathology.

Another caution that must be observed is related to the regulations in some school systems that prohibit anyone except the school physician, and possibly the school nurse, from conducting any test or examination that requires the placement of any instrument, including a tongue blade, inside a pupil's mouth. Under these circumstances, of course, no effort should be made to view the vocal folds, but most of the other vital structures and their functions can be observed without putting anything into the mouth except light.

EXAMINATION OF THE ORGANS OF SPEECH. After completing the formal assessment and recording of the voice, the patient is taken to a room or an area of the interviewing office where equipment is arranged for the examination.

The examiner must at this time wash his hands carefully before he approaches the task of viewing the mechanism used in speaking. Subsequently, the subject and examiner sit facing each other and the three-phase examination begins. The first part, observation of external features, includes the noting of scars or other unusual features on the head, face, and neck, and the habitual posture of the lips, including the presence of mouth breathing. Most of these items will have been observed informally during the preceding interview and voice recording. In the formal observation session questions can be asked about the scars to learn their causes, when they occurred, and whether or not there is any relationship between them and the voice problem. If mouth breathing is evident, there should be careful observations of the rest positions of the lips and their size. Chronic breathing through the mouth lessens the activity of the upper lip and causes it to become shorter, thereby exposing the upper teeth except when an effort is made to bring the lips together. Concurrently, the lower lip becomes large and pendant, and the mentalis muscle is excessively developed through its use in elevating the lower lip. The evidence of excessive development of the mentalis muscle is the presence of a prominent muscular "button" below the lip on the front of the chin. Chronic mouth breathing indicates restricted or blocked nasal passages and suggests enlarged adenoidal tissue, an allergic reaction, polyps or other tumorous developments, or occlusion from an injury to the nose. To check on the mobility of the facial muscles, the patient should be asked to pucker his lips and then to smile broadly. This procedure reveals general control and symmetry of the face. It is evident that the facial muscles are not directly involved in voice production, but if asymmetrical movements are present, they may signal a paralysis of some sort and consequently alert the examiner for subsequent observations of other structures.

The second phase of the examination of the mechanism is directed to the mouth and oropharynx. First, observe the evenness, color, and general attractiveness of the teeth. This step has particular significance in the case of girls and young women, since they sometimes attempt to hide unattractive teeth by keeping the mouth relatively closed and holding the upper lip over the teeth. Embarrassment of this type may contribute to articulatory problems, social withdrawal, and inadequate voice production. The teeth should also be seen in occlusion to note the bite relationships of the upper and lower anterior teeth. Malocclusions may also have detrimental cosmetic, articulatory, psychological, and social effects. If articulatory disorders are observed, this fact should be recorded and considered in therapy. The fact that persons often have articulatory problems along with voice disorders needs to be remembered.

When observing the teeth it is desirable to instruct the patient to open his mouth and, while directing the light from a flashlight or concave mirror onto the back teeth, to note the general condition of the teeth and the type of dental care that has existed. Persons with caries reflect lack of attention and possibly an attitude concerning self or family that could be significant in any therapeutic effort for voice.

Examination of the mouth should continue with attention directed to the tongue. First, the patient should be asked to protrude his tongue as far as possible along the mid-line. Usually the tests of tongue control and mobility are carried out most easily when the examiner simply says, "Do this," and then protrudes his own tongue so the patient can imitate the maneuver. While the tongue is out, the patient should be told to curl the tip upward toward the nose, downward toward the chin, and from side to side several times. If the point of the tongue deviates to one side or the other when it is protruded and if there is extreme effort needed to move it laterally, a paralysis can be suspected. Next, ask the patient to say a series of "la-la-la" sounds while the examiner observes the lifting and lowering of the tongue. If the movement is sluggish or if the point of the tongue draws somewhat laterally when it is lifted, there is additional reason to suspect neural involvement. The "la" sequence should be followed by the instruction to say "kitty-kitty-kitty" or "Tinker-toy—Tinker-toy" precisely and at a moderately rapid rate. The combinations of sounds in these utterances require coordination of all of the tongue muscles as the back and front of that organ are alternately lifted. If there is slowness or more serious difficulty with the rapid sound sequences, a weakness or paralysis may be suspected.

An effort should also be made to assess the size of the tongue. If it appears to overflow its space as it rests on the floor of the mouth or if there are prominent serrations along its lateral margins that mark the positions of the teeth, the tongue can be classified as large. This factor probably has no significance in speech if the articulation of speech sounds is adequate, but if the voice is also somewhat hoarse, symptoms of thyroid imbalance should be investigated in the subsequent case history interview.

After observing the tongue, the light should be directed upward to note the shape, color, scars, and other atypical features of both the hard and soft palates and the mobility of the latter. If the previous voice assessment indicated excessive nasal resonance, the palate requires special attention. The height and contour of the palatal vault should be noted, as well as the color of the mucosa. If the vault is particularly high and the voice somewhat denasal, there is a possibility that the high palate has reduced the size of the nasal space and partially occluded the airway. If the color of the mucous membrane, particularly over the alveolar ridge and velum, is pale, anemia should be suspected and the possibility of referral considered. In contrast, if the small blood vessels of the soft palate are dilated to give it a general redness, there is a strong implication that the patient is smoking heavily, has an allergy, or is suffering a "cold." While the examiner is observing the velum, he should note the movement of that structure when the patient is instructed to say an *ah* or *eh* sound. The soft palate should swing upward and backward quickly and symmetrically on both sides. If it does not move or if it draws laterally as it lifts, some paralysis can be suspected. If the patient has exhibited a hypernasality, an impairment of velar movement would be anticipated. However, if the palate lifts symmetrically and quickly but hypernasality persists, the presumption is either that the velopharyngeal structures are not large enough to effect a closure—that is, the nasopharynx is relatively too deep or the velum is too short—or that there is a submucal cleft. Where there is a double, or bifid, uvula, the latter presumption is the more probable. The presence of scars anywhere on the palate should lead to exploratory questions about them.

Observation logically shifts from the velum proper to the faucial region and the palatine tonsils. The presence or absence, size, and color of these structures should be noted, and when the history interview is resumed, questions about recent medical care should be explored. A medical evaluation should be required if there has been a history of throat discomfort and if the individual has not had recent medical assistance.

Additional observation in the faucial and pharyngeal regions should reveal the presence of any scar tissue in the tonsillar sites or surrounding areas and the uniformity of the posterior border of the velum. If there are extensive scars or if one side of the velum is higher than the other, the valving action of the structure may be impaired and cause nasality. Occasionally the posterior wall of the pharynx can be seen to slide laterally when the patient attempts to close the velopharyngeal valve. This behavior indicates a unilateral paralysis of a pharyngeal constrictor muscle, a condition that usually is combined with a comparable impairment of the palatal musculature. The involvement of both groups of muscles increases the severity of the speech problem.

At this point attention can be directed to the nasal passages. The patient should be asked to hum an easy *m* sound to note more carefully the nature of the nasal resonance. While the tone is being prolonged, the examiner should press the ala of one nostril to occlude the passage and to note the change of voice quality. The same procedure should be followed for the opposite side. If partial or complete stoppages are present, questions may reveal how long they have existed and their relationships to allergies, colds, injuries, or sinus infections. Attention to the patency of the nasal passages is particularly important when the voice sounds denasal.

The third phase of the examination of the speech mechanism is the study of the interior of the larynx. The type of voice noted during the assessment will determine the primary focus of the observation, but an evaluation of the entire structure should be made. To accomplish this task systematically, it is suggested that the sequence as outlined below be followed.

An attempt should be made first to see the vocal folds, since they are the source of phonatory problems and since the length of time for viewing may be brief, due to the patient's reactions. Factors to be noted are color, size, similarity of movements in adduction and abduction, the presence of asymmetries in size or position, and circumscribed enlargements, such as nodules, edematous areas, papillomas, cysts, and the like. It is important that the vocal cords be viewed throughout their entire lengths, including the anterior commissure, and that the location and estimate of size of any abnormality be noted. The vibratory patterns of the folds are not visible to the unaided eye, but the implications of paralysis, tumors, and other diseases, as revealed in ultra high speed films, have been discussed previously, and insightful predictions of the effects of any observed deviations can be made.

The next structures to be viewed in a logical sequence are the ventricular folds, aryepiglottic folds, the arytenoid cartilages, and the epiglottis. The actual and relative sizes and colors of these parts should be noted and a judgment made of their possible influence on the voice. It is also desirable to view the areas immediately external to the larynx, such as the pyriform sinuses, the pharyngeal mucosa, and the vallecula between the epiglottis and tongue, to note any condition that would justify medical referral.

A PROCEDURE FOR VISUAL INSPECTION OF THE LARYNX. The location of the larynx and the physiological constraints associated with attempts to observe it constitute the problems that must be managed for successful visualization of the vocal folds. It is apparent that the larynx is situated where it cannot be viewed without the aid of an instrument; its vertical axis is approximately at right angles to the anterior-posterior dimension of the mouth; it is in a dark area that must be especially illuminated if it is to be seen; and the normal faucial and pharyngeal reflexes tend to reject the presence of an instrument in these areas.

The equipment needed for visualizing the larynx can vary considerably in elaborateness, but the basic essentials that will serve the speech pathologist are relatively simple. There should be two straight chairs that can be arranged to face each other; a small table or desk on which a few instruments can be placed; a bright light, the source of which may be either an ordinary 100 or 200 watt lamp, or a "bulls eye" examination bulb that is frosted except for a clear circular area on one side, or a regular 35 mm slide projector; a physician's $3\frac{1}{2}$ inch concave head mirror and supporting head band; an assortment of laryngeal mirrors of varying sizes, including numbers 3, 4, 5, and 6, which increase progressively from $\frac{3}{4}$ to $1\frac{1}{8}$ inches in diameter; a small spirit lamp for heating the laryngeal mirrors; and a few sterile gauze squares, 2" x 2" or slightly larger, for holding the patient's tongue. The illumination lamp should be placed so that it is near the side of the patient's head and above the level of his ear. The side on which it is placed is a matter of the examiner's choice, but it is customary for right handed persons to place the lamp on the patient's right side to avoid the possibility of the examiner's right hand and arm coming between the light source and the concave head mirror, thereby shading the mirror.

The speech pathologist is not privileged to use an anaesthetic in the mouth and pharynx of the person being examined to reduce sensitivity and thereby to simplify the procedure. Consequently, it is essential that the technique be developed carefully and perfected, so that the larynx can be viewed as completely as necessary without discomfort to the patient. It is presumed in this discussion that the assessment of the oral structures, as described above, has occurred immediately prior to the examination of the larynx. The subject has become adjusted to the speech pathologist and usually cooperates without hesitation.

To view the vocal folds, the examiner should ask the patient to sit erect and to lean forward from the hips with his back straight and his chin thrust slightly forward. A clean laryngeal mirror is warmed over the spirit lamp to a temperature slightly above that of the body, and the amount of heat tested by touching the metal case of the mirror to the back of the hand near the thumb. The subject is then requested to open his mouth and to protrude his tongue. One of the gauze squares is placed over the upper and lower surfaces of the extended part of the tongue, and the examiner grasps that structure firmly with his thumb and forefinger and the intervening gauze. The thumb should rest on the under surface, the forefinger on the upper side, and the middle finger by vertical extension rests against the patient's upper lateral incisor tooth. This latter adjustment helps to hold the patient's mouth open.

When the mouth is in this position, the warm laryngeal mirror, which is held like a pencil, is moved back through the mouth as the patient is instructed to prolong an [ε] sound at a relatively high pitch. The mirror should not touch the tongue and ordinarily goes back to the uvula, at which point the light can be reflected downward past the base of the tongue to the epiglottis. A small adjustment of the mirror to move it deeper into the pharynx brings the arytenoid area into view and also the interior of the larynx. A limited rotation of the mirror handle or a slight shift upward or downward may improve the illumination in the larynx and thereby improve the observation of the vocal cords.

The [ε] sound is recommended because it is produced with the tongue in a relatively low, fronted position, which represents a compromise between the widest mouth position and the largest opening into the larynx. The vowel [ɑ], which requires the lowest tongue position in the mouth, is made with the back of the tongue retracted into the pharynx, which presses the epiglottis backward and obscures the interior of the larynx. In contrast, the vowel [i] causes the epiglottis to be in its most forward position, thereby opening the larynx maximally, but this vowel requires a high, forward tongue position which obstructs the view of the laryngeal mirror when it is in the pharynx. The intermediate [ε] is an effective compromise, but occasionally when the anterior parts of the vocal cords are hidden by the epiglottis, it is helpful to instruct the patient to try to utter a high piched [i]. His attempt will not produce an [i] if the tongue is held down, but the epiglottis is moved forward as part of the attempt, and the anterior portion of the larynx often comes into view.

Usually the vocal folds can be seen while the initial [ε] sound is being produced, but, regardless, the patient eventually exhausts his breath supply and must inhale. This maneuver causes the vocal folds to abduct and gives the examiner an opportunity to see their margins and also to look into the trachea. In most subjects an alternating series of inhalations and productions of [ɛ] or [i] sounds can be accomplished to provide a good view of the various structures to assess their color, abduction, and adduction, as well as any tumors or other abnormal developments.

Most persons tolerate a mirror in the pharynx and permit a view of the larynx. However, there are a few who, because their reflexes are genuinely sensitive or because they are too apprehensive of the procedure to cooperate, cannot be examined without the use of an anaesthetic. The condition of the larynx in these individuals and the possible causes of a phonatory problem must be determined primarily from a laryngologist's report and the case history.

By the time the survey of the speech mechanism has been completed in the sequential evaluation of the voice disorder, the speech pathologist will have recognized and described the voice problem, he will know something of its history, and he will have a more or less positive concept of its immediate cause. In fact, it is entirely possible that an organic problem and its influence on the voice may be so clearly established that additional probing is unnecessary at this time. However, the listening, looking, and limited questioning conducted previously may not reveal enough of the etiology to form a rational therapy; consequently, additional searching must be carried on. When this situation exists, the speech pathologist resumes the history interview, to explore questions suggested during the examination of the structures and to inquire into potentially relevant factors of development, health, family, and environment.

DEVELOPMENT OF THE INDIVIDUAL AND HIS SPEECH

If a voice disorder has existed since infancy or if the circumstances related to its initiation are vague, it is desirable to determine, if possible, whether the disorder is hereditary, congenital, acquired through vocal abuse, or is the result of paralysis, tumor, or other disease. An approach to these possible sources can be made through answers to the following questions: Was there anything unusual about the birth? Was breathing normal from the start? Was the breathing noisy during sleep or at other times? Was the cry loud and vigorous or was it weak? Was the voice low-pitched or hoarse? Was there much crying and screaming in the first month of life, or was he remembered as a quiet or "good baby"? When did he sit alone? When did he begin to walk? When did he use his first words purposely? Did he ever lose his voice? When and under what circumstances? When did the change of voice occur? Was there anything unusual about it?

Replies that indicate a deviation from normal at birth or in the developmental schedules require supplemental questions about learning and health.

Health History

The voice is a sensitive indicator of the current state of health of an individual, his emotional stability, and the relative structural condition of his larynx. In attempting to determine the source of a voice disorder when the source is not clearly evident, it is essential that at least the following aspects of the health history be explored.

INJURIES AND SURGICAL PROCEDURES. Injuries or surgical procedures affecting the regions of the head, neck, or chest may, through involvement of the nervous system or organs used in speaking, interfere with normal voice production. The following types of questions are useful: Was there an accident or injury preceding the recognition of the voice problem? Was any type of surgery performed? What was the reason for it and what structures were altered? Was speaking affected? Was breathing affected? Was swallowing affected? Were there ever any severe blows to the head, nose, or throat?

ILLNESS AND DISEASE. The potential significance of localized disease, such as tumors in the larynx and paralysis of the velum, and systemic disorders, such as allergic response and anemia, were reviewed in the preceding chapter. Systematic exploratory questions, based on such information, may reveal either reasons for referral or clues to successful voice therapy. The following questions have proved to be useful when used appropriately in relation to vocal symptoms and other case history information. Was there an illness during the two to three months before the voice disorder was observed? What was it called? How severe was it? Was it treated by a medical doctor? Was there anything unusual about the convalescence? Has the illness been associated in any way with the voice? Was a tooth extracted or other dental work performed a short time before the voice disorder became apparent? Which of the following diseases has the individual had: measles, mumps, scarlet fever, diphtheria, poliomyelitis, bronchitis, or undiagnosed high fever? When did each reported disease occur and how severe was it? Has the individual ever had any convulsions? When and what caused them? Have they been controlled? Is medication being used currently?

Has anemia ever been present? When? Was it treated medically? Is there now, or has there ever been, allergic sensitivity to any foods? What types? How was or is the condition controlled? Does the individual have hay fever, rose fever, or other similar reactions? Has there ever been a thyroid problem or other metabolic disturbance? What were the symptoms? Was it treated medically?

What medications have been or are being taken more or less regularly? What is the purpose? Does the individual use tranquilizers? How frequently and for what purpose? Is aspirin used frequently? How often and for what purpose? Has any type of hormone injection or medication ever been used? Why was it prescribed?

HEARING AND EAR PROBLEMS. The individual with a hearing loss or a history of ear problems may be unable to regulate the loudness or pitch of his voice. Questions should inquire about hearing ability, history of ear ache, draining ear, and injuries to the ears. Such inquiries should follow hearing tests, particularly when the audiogram shows a hearing loss. An audiometric examination should be conducted regularly for all persons with voice disorders.

Environmental Factors

Questions about the environment are based on the presumption that voice disorders may be developed through imitation; by vigorous vocal use in reaction to, and competition with, associates; or as a consequence of vocal demands at work, recreation, school, and home. The following questions are useful in exploring the environmental situation: Are there any known voice or speech defects in the immediate family or among other relatives, including aunts, uncles, grandparents, and cousins? Has the patient ever lived with or been associated with persons having voice disorders? Is his voice similar to that of anyone else in the family? How do members of the family refer to the voice problem when talking about it among themselves? How noisy is his place of work? Does he have any noisy hobbies?

Assessment of the Need for Additional Information

When a direct assessment of a voice disorder, combined with a survey of the history of the individual as it relates to the vocal problem, fails to provide an adequate diagnosis, additional information may be needed. Assistance can be obtained from such other specialists as otolaryngologists, neurologists, endocrinologists, pediatricians, psychologists, psychiatrists, or others as deemed necessary. Such referrals delay the completion of an evaluation, but an inadequate diagnosis is a poor starting point for therapy. Frequently such delays can be avoided by requesting at least an otologic and laryngologic evaluation by an otolaryngologist prior to the diagnostic session for the voice.

When a referral is made to one of the medical specialties, the speech pathologist should clarify the purpose of the referral and indicate the kinds of services needed. If the patient is to be turned over completely to the physician for treatment and management, this fact should be stated, and any subsequent introduction of voice therapy must receive the approval of the physician. However, if circumstances indicate that an additional opinion is needed—for example, on the nature and effect of an allergic reaction—the referring request should be for a consultative opinion. The latter will enable the speech pathologist, or the team of specialists with whom he works, to reach a proper decision.

Summary of Findings and Diagnosis

The pertinent data need to be brought together and a diagnosis or tentative diagnosis developed. The significance of certain factors can be noted and a unified concept constructed most effectively in conference with others who have also seen the patient. However, when one works alone, one must play multiple roles and be doubly certain of his evaluation of the potentially significant items. The speech pathologist should realize that diagnosis and evaluation are continuous processes that accompany therapy, and that there should be no compulsion to reach a final decision in a difficult case if the data gathered in a relatively brief period do not justify it.

Recommendations

Where possible, and it is usually possible, positive statements based on the findings should be made about management of the voice disorder as a guide to the patient and to the person charged with therapy. These particular recommendations customarily state whether or not voice therapy is indicated; whether or not a referral is advised; the nature of certain changes in vocal usage that must be introduced; the changes in the environment that should be instituted; and the date for a reevaluation if voice therapy is not recommended or is to be carried on by a person at some other location.

Clinician's Assessment of the Diagnostic Session

Some diagnostic interviews and test procedures progress smoothly and the necessary information is obtained easily and efficiently. Conversely, there are occasions in which great effort is expended in eliciting replies and in obtaining cooperation from patient or parents. Such factors may be important in the evaluation of the individual and his problem, but they may not be apparent in the usual reporting procedures. Since the validity of diagnostic findings may vary in relation to the relationship between the patient and the diagnostic situation and since many clinicians may review the diagnostic report over a period of time, it is essential that the elements influencing the situation be made apparent. To accomplish this objective the following scale should be completed for each patient. Check marks should be placed along the continuum between the contrasting terms, at points representing the clinician's evaluation of the patient's attitude or response.

talkative	_____	inarticulate
assertive	_____	shy
relaxed, at ease	_____	tense, apprehensive
alert, enthusiastic	_____	apathetic
cheerful	_____	gloomy
arrogant	_____	humble
conventional	_____	individualistic, eccentric
fastidious	_____	coarse
formal	_____	informal
friendly	_____	hostile

THE PRESENCE OF VOICE DEFECTS THAT ARE CAUSED BY ORGANIC DIS-orders indicates the existence of some type of alteration in the vocal structures. This observation recognizes also that voice therapy for such voice problems normally incorporates certain medical specialties in addition to speech pathology; that is, vocal rehabilitation is the proper concern of several professional groups. Each specialty has certain responsibilities and obligations to the person with a voice defect and to the associated professions. This relationship necessitates cooperative effort for the benefit of the patient, genuine team work in which the speech pathologist must accept his full responsibility.

In an effort to delineate the professional obligations and to emphasize the facets of vocal therapy, the following discussion will

6 *therapeutic procedures*

touch on (1) the several types of therapeutic procedure that are available; (2) the professional worker who is responsible for each kind of therapy; (3) the etiologies and underlying presumptions that provide the rationale for the various kinds of therapy; (4) the changes that are expected to result from the procedures; and (5) the specific therapeutic measures through which the desired results are achieved.

TYPES OF THERAPEUTIC PROCEDURE

Therapy for organically related voice disorders encompasses, in varying proportions, three principal types of remedial procedure: restoration of the vocal mechanism to its maximum possible efficiency; modification of the relationships between the individual and his environment; and alterations of the individual's behavior, including both his habits of vocal use and his thinking. The first of these therapeutic objectives is composed primarily of procedures that can be done for, or to, the individual with his minimal active participation. The second may or may not require the patient's participation, depending upon the type of environmental changes that are desired. The third approach requires, and its success depends upon, the cooperation and active participation by the patient. In some instances only one of these procedures is needed, in others two or three. The therapies may be employed separately or in combination and in various sequences. The therapeutic regimen of choice is based upon patient need and feasibility.

PROFESSIONAL RESPONSIBILITY

When a defective voice is caused by an abnormal structure or impaired organ that can be corrected or improved by surgical procedures, medication, x-ray, or some comparable treatment, the initial therapy, and sometimes the entire vocal restoration, is accomplished by persons in the medical profession. When voice disorders are developed or maintained as the result of detrimental environmental conditions, the responsibility for initiating and pursuing the necessary modifications rests with the speech pathologist, the physician, the social worker, and perhaps the counselor. Parents also may improve the environment to benefit a child; an employer can modify the working conditions for an employee; and the patient himself may alter the factors in his surroundings to reduce those conditions that contribute detrimentally to his voice production. When the medical therapy that is necessary has been instituted and the required environmental changes effected, the process of direct voice therapy, which is prescribed and guided by the speech pathologist and learned by the patient, can be developed.

An alternate way of indicating the responsibility of the speech pathologist in the rehabilitation of the patient with an organic voice disorder is to observe that the speech pathologist cannot perform surgery or practice the other medical arts; instead, he must use those therapeutic techniques appropriate to his profession. These procedures encompass the range of reeducative activities that extend from the modification of vocal behavior to the alteration of environment and the improvement of both physical and mental hygiene. These techniques may be employed after medical treatment, concurrently with such treatment or independently when medical intervention is not needed.

If the speech pathologist understands the kinds of organic change that are possible in the vocal mechanism and the ways in which these deviations can affect the voice and if he recognizes the range of therapeutic procedure available to him, then he can institute a rational therapy. Unfortunately, since the cause and effect relationships have not been precisely determined in many problems and since therapeutic measures are frequently not subject to predictable results from patient to patient, the selection and application of specific procedures is determined by the judgment of the therapist; consequently, the practice of voice therapy is still largely an art.

MEDICAL THERAPY

Structural abnormalities and organic variations in the larynx and resonators may cause abnormal vocal sound. Organic variations in the larynx encompass such conditions as congenital anomalies, fractures, dislocations, cysts, paralyses, excess mucus, edema, and both malignant and benign tumors, the most common of the latter being polyps, nodules, and papillomas. Organic changes in the resonators include more or less complete occlusion of the vocal space, changes in the character of the mucosa within the upper respiratory tract, and impairment in the capacity of the velopharyngeal valve to function adequately. Maximum improvement of the impaired vocal mechanism is desirable as a basis for the development or restoration of more normal vocal sound. Many of the problems can be remedied or improved by surgery or medication.

Results to Be Expected from Medical Therapy

It can be expected that the correction of the anomalies and the removal of the offending tumors and other irregularities will improve glottal closure and restore the vocal folds to a more flexible condition, thereby enhancing their ability to vibrate and to interrupt the air flow at the glottis. Appropriate medication can be expected to influence the voice favorably by reduction of swelling in the vocal folds, pharynx, and nose; improvement of conditions at the cricoarytenoid joints; normalization of mucosal secretion; increase of blood supply to the muscles; and improvement of neural functioning. The vocal improvement can be in loudness, quality, or pitch, depending upon the effect of the underlying impairment.

Therapeutic Techniques and Measures Employed in Medical Therapy

The means used by the surgeon and physician to accomplish these various changes include, selectively and appropriately, excision, reconstructive surgery, teflon injection, and radiation therapy. Other

> 37   Teflon is being used frequently in rehabilitation for vocal fold paralysis. What is the function of this substance and how is it employed? The article by Arnold (2) is quite instructive.

medical treatment employs medicaments for the treatment of localized disease and for the management of such systemic involvements as allergic reactions, anemia, and metabolic disturbances. Additional therapy often recommended by the physician encompasses protection against airborne irritating pollutants and the elimination of both smoking and alcohol.

ENVIRONMENTAL THERAPY

Medical treatment and vocal reeducation rarely accomplish any lasting improvement in a defective voice so long as the client lives or works in an environment that is responsible for vocal abuse or damage to the vocal organs. Most persons have not learned how to use their voices without abusing the structures, and many of them work and live where shouting and excessive speaking are commonplace. These patterns of vocal use create changes in both the surface and deeper structures of the larynx that can impair vocal fold vibration.

Some environments contain irritants or allergens that adversely effect the mucosa of the respiratory tract and consequently cause vocal problems. These substances may exert their effects on the voice directly through the reactive swelling of the mucous membrane and excessive mucus secretion, or they may create changes in the membrane which, when combined with vocal abuse, exaggerate the effects of both the irritants and the traumatic phonation.

Results to Be Expected from Environmental Therapy

When attention to the environment lessens shouting and other abuse, there will be a reduction or elimination of vocal nodules, chronic laryngitis, contact ulcer, and other problems that may be caused by vocal misuse. Reduction of irritants and allergens can be expected to allow the mucosa to return to a healthier condition and thereby to be capable of more normal vibration. A further benefit of environmental improvement is the favorable effect these changes have as support for direct voice therapy.

Procedures for Improving the Vocal Environment

Occasionally a patient can modify his speaking requirements in his various environments through his own efforts after he understands the relationships between his voice and his surroundings. More frequently, however, it is necessary for the speech pathologist, physician, social worker, or counselor to become involved with the environment and to provide the actual leadership for seeking the necessary changes. This procedure requires interviews with parents and teachers if the problem exists in a child, or with employers and families when the disorder is present in adults. Where sufficient insight and understanding exist, adjustments are usually not difficult to accomplish, but when the patient considers his voice to be relatively unimportant or when the employment situation cannot be altered, the chance for environmental change is remote. The conscientious speech pathologist will rarely feel justified in refusing to work with an individual primarily on the basis of a detrimental environmental situation, but he must realize that the therapeutic process is more or less jeopardized.

There are at least two objectives of interviews with parents and other members of a child's family. Basically, the initial purpose is to obtain reduction in the amount of use and loudness of the child's voice when he is at home and at play. Where possible without nagging, he can be reminded to speak more softly and to speak less frequently. With many children eight years of age and older the response is favorable and progress is made. Of course, the speech clinician provides explanations for the procedure and strongly supports the child's efforts. However, with the younger child this approach is rarely successful because he lacks the capacity to avoid vigorous verbal competition with other children in the family and perhaps even with his parents. In such a world the child who remains quiet is handicapped, and from his standpoint he finds it more desirable to live with a hoarse voice and vocal nodules than as a disadvantaged member of his family.

The second objective of conferences with the family is related to and supplements the purpose for the first but involves the family more and the patient less. This objective is to help the parents create and maintain a quieter household environment. If one or both parents can be brought to realize that there is excessive talk and that this is contributing to the child's problem, such behavior can sometimes be changed. When quieter voices are used by the parents and disciplinary measures are employed that do not include shouting, substantial improvement in household management often results.

One method that usually helps a family realize the amount of speaking done, and thereby contributes to improvement of the vocal environment, is the establishment of a period of 10–15 minutes after the evening meal (or some prefer 5 minutes during the meal) during which no one is allowed to say anything except in an emergency. Those who break the silence are required to pay a penalty. This practice causes many persons to become aware for the first time that they do indeed talk more than they thought they did.

Modification of the environment of an adult who has a voice problem is usually accomplished through direct work with him. Discussions about laryngeal trauma and its consequences provide insight for the patient into such vocal abuses as excessive speaking, shouting at sporting events, loud singing, and loud talking in noisy working situations. As a consequence, the individual arrives at an understanding of what he must do to improve his voice. If his employment environment cannot be modified, he may be able to change his manner of speaking by using an amplifying system to compensate for the noise. He may also be able to use ear wardens to reduce the effects of the surrounding noise and thereby lessen the tendency to shout when attempting to speak in the noisy environment.

The place where an individual lives or works may be detrimental to the voice, not only because it encourages vocal abuse but also because the air in it contains pollen, dust, or other pollutants that irritate the linings of the airway. Frequently, the regular use of air conditioners, air filters, face masks, or humidifiers can lessen the detrimental effects sufficiently to reduce or eliminate the problem. In rare instances it may be necessary for an individual to move his place of residence or occupation to escape from the environmental

DIRECT VOCAL REHABILITATION

The two preceding types of therapy presumed that the voice will improve if certain detrimental conditions are removed or altered. Those approaches allow the person with the disorder to remain relatively passive. In contrast, the third form of therapy, the modification of the patterns that produce the undesirable sounds, requires direct work with and active participation by the patient. To affect a change in the voice, there must be a change in the manner of voice production; the individual must learn new or modified vocal habits. Improving such habits is a learning process, whether the problem is organically or functionally based, and the procedures applied to one are frequently the same as those used with the other. This apparent commonality of therapeutic techniques in organic and functional disorders tends to confuse those who do not recognize the difference between therapeutic methods and therapy. Vocal therapy is individualized; it is composed of vocal reeducation methods or techniques that are combined in uniquely special patterns to suit the needs of the patient. A specific procedure might be used with two patients to accomplish different results with each.

The modification of habituated behavior, which is often complicated by disease or structural change, encompasses many interrelated procedures, the most common of which are vocal training, relaxation, listening ("ear training"), regulation of breath pressure, posture, physical hygiene, and mental hygiene. The presumptions and expected results of each of these aspects of therapy should be reviewed individually.

Rationale for Vocal Training and the Expected Results of the Procedure

There is considerable clinical evidence that organic changes in the larynx or in the resonators which result from surgery or disease and which cause voice disorders can often be modified beneficially by vocal exercises and special attention to compensatory adjustments. There is also evidence that laryngeal disorders stemming from vocal trauma, including such problems as vocal nodules, contact ulcer, and other changes, respond to vocal training. Reducing or eliminating vocal abuse can be accomplished by substituting nontraumatizing voice production. One means of developing the desired new vocal usage is through vocal reeducation.

38   Are there any vocal reeducation techniques that are common to the therapeutic procedures for vocal nodules as presented by Brodnitz (11) and Greene (39)?

Direct training of the voice can be expected to produce a more pleasant sounding voice in which inappropriate pitch can be brought toward the normal, deviations in loudness can be reduced, and abnormal quality can be made more nearly normal. A vocal training program should also establish the more efficient use of the larynx and the resonators. Efficiency in voice production means less effort to produce the sounds, greater flexibility of the voice, less effortful production of loud sounds, and the increased clarity of the sound, that is, reduced hoarseness or other phonatory or resonance deviations.

As suggested above, training an individual to use his voice without traumatizing the structures can usually create a condition in which vocal nodules, contact ulcer, and similar problems will recede or disappear. Where permanent organic changes in the larynx exist, vocal training is compensatory. It is directed toward developing the most acceptable voice possible and, where the sound is abnormal, helping the patient to live with it.

Methods and Procedures in Voice Training

Occasionally, voice therapy includes a period of vocal silence while healing occurs following surgery or when minimum laryngeal use for some other organic reason is necessary. However, sooner or later phonation must be introduced if reeducation is to occur. Such phonation is part of what is included in "voice training," but the term encompasses all phonation done for a purpose, from sung sounds and vocal gymnastics to spoken sentences and paragraphs.

> 39 Why does Brodnitz question the use of a period of vocal silence in the therapy for contact ulcer and vocal nodules? Note what he says in (12).

It is not the province of this book to offer specific exercises or drills, but there are a few fundamental principles that govern vocal reeducation. When the patient presents himself for therapy, he is capable of speaking and of producing sounds at a certain level of excellence. He cannot be expected at that time to perform beyond his existing capacity. Consequently, therapy begins with what can be done best and progresses from that point. It is necessary to discover the vowel, the pitch, and the loudness at which the individual produces vocal sounds most effectively. If this production agrees with the known condition of the larynx and does not threaten to abuse the structures, then these sounds constitute the start of direct vocal rehabilitation.

Usually all exercising in the initial stages of voice therapy is done with minimum loudness and for short periods; excessive muscle tension of the laryngeal and pharyngeal muscles must be avoided. A slightly breathy voice is often desirable to introduce relatively easy, effortless phonation in the early stages of therapy. When single sounds are sung or spoken, there should be considerable pitch variation. Excessive prolongation of tones or use of one pitch should be avoided in the early stages of therapy. Progressive, controlled pitch changes are produced by gradual increases and decreases of muscle contraction in the larynx, adjustments that tend to reduce the random vibratory variability that causes vocal roughness.

Learning to change pitch voluntarily constitutes an important stage in control of vocalization, which is the focus of vocal exercises. Another aid in control is the intentional modification of vocal quality or timbre. The breathy voice referred to above is one of the easiest to achieve and is a good one to practice in conjunction with different vocal pitches. Other voluntary voice differences are hypernasality, in which much of the sound and breath are allowed to escape through the nose, and the opposite condition, denasality, in which a "cold in the head" quality is produced. The patient should be encouraged to imitate the voices of professional actors or friends when these efforts are not detrimental. Such vocal types are not recommended as desirable kinds of voice to use; they are suggested as exercises to enable the patient to gain control over his vocal organs. He should learn to produce various vocal qualities at will, to enable him to speak with a satisfactory voice that is itself not detrimental or traumatic to the vocal mechanism. Vocal exercises of all types should be combined in therapy with the other procedures that were indicated previously.

The basic presumption or justification for selected vocal exercises is that they can sometimes modify phonation or resonance characteristics to compensate for surgical alteration, disease, or detrimental habits. Where structural modification lessens or prevents the possibility of a normal voice, vocal exercises may lead to a stronger voice, less effort in voice production, or more pleasant vocal sound. Vocal exercises of various types are also used as a direct remedy for organic problems that are related to vocal abuse, such as vocal nodules and contact ulcer. In fact, it has been demonstrated that these organic problems are rarely corrected unless vocal abuse is eliminated.

A Rationale for Relaxation and Notations of the Expected Results

The use of relaxation exercises in vocal therapy is based on the following presumptions: (1) that several voice disorders are caused by, or are maintained by, excessive contraction of the adductory muscles; (2) that this muscular imbalance can be reduced or eliminated by relaxation procedures; (3) that relaxation will facilitate efficient voice production and will reduce the condition that contributes to the formation of vocal nodules and other traumatic disorders; and (4) that physical relaxation can be learned. The development of the capacity to relax is expected to improve the vocal tone, to reduce vocal trauma, and generally to allow the vocal folds to be adjusted in relation to each other and internally for maximum vibrational efficiency.

Method and Procedures in Relaxation

Relaxation, as used in vocal rehabilitation, refers not to flaccidity, which is sometimes associated with the term, but rather to coordination. Relaxation implies efficiency of movement resulting from the balanced interplay of the groups of opposing muscles. If certain muscles contract when they should be relaxing, there is an imbalance, energy is wasted, adjustments of the organs of speech are accomplished only with effort, and the result is less than needed.

Excessive tension in antagonistic muscle groups of the larynx can cause a range of responses from clumsiness, that is, slight incoordination, to tremor and spasticity. When these forms of behavior are related to voice production, they cause variable laryngeal adjustments and uncertainty of vocal initiation, tremulousness, or excessive closure of the glottis, resulting in such vocal disorders as intermittent phonation, spastic dysphonia, harshness, roughness, or aphonia. Persistent phonation when there is excessive tension in the laryngeal muscles may lead to vocal nodules, contact ulcer, chronic inflammation of laryngeal tissue, or thickened mucosa. It follows that relaxation is essential in the relief of such vocal and laryngeal problems.

40   Note the insightful and practical discussion of relaxation by Van Riper and Irwin (88:307–11).

Resonance disorders are also closely associated with imbalance in muscle contraction, particularly within the pharyngeal area. Distortion in nasal resonance, resulting from inadequate adjustment of the velopharyngeal valve, and the over emphasis of high partials, resulting from contraction of the pharyngeal constrictor muscles, represent types of distortion that may be present.

Training in relaxation focuses on (1) the voluntary muscles of the body; (2) the organs of speech; and (3) such emotional reactions as anxiety, worry, and anger. Each emphasis is related to the others, each is necessary, and all may require diligent concentration over considerable periods of time.

RELAXATION OF THE SKELETAL MUSCLES. Purposive relaxation of the voluntary muscles of the body can be accomplished by either of two commonly used techniques. One of these is sometimes referred to as the "suggestion procedure," the other as "progressive relaxation." In the former a sensation is imagined as a substitute or replacement for the feeling of excessive muscle contraction. The individual learns the "suggestion technique" while either sitting in a comfortable chair or lying down, and imagining a sensation of heaviness spreading progressively, slowly, and methodically through his feet, legs, hands, arms, neck, back, abdomen, chest, face, and head. Frequent practice sessions are often necessary to accomplish positive results that can be extended beyond the quiet practice period.

The second procedure, "progressive relaxation," was presented originally by Edmund Jacobson, M.D. (49 and 50), who used it with patients having various chronic illnesses. The basis of the technique is the recognition and localization by the patient of muscles in contraction, and the voluntary relaxation of the contraction. The method of identifying muscle contraction is by resistance to motion; for example, the patient attempts to flex an arm while the clinician resists the movement. While this activity is being performed, the patient observes the sensation of contraction in the muscles of the upper arm and then notes the difference when he ceases his effort. When the individual learns to identify muscle contraction, he can usually release it voluntarily. As skill is achieved through practice with the skeletal muscles, the ability is transferred to less easily identified and controlled muscles. Some of these are in the oral, laryngeal, and pharyngeal areas.

RELAXATION OF THE MUSCLES USED IN SPEAKING. Relaxation of the organs of speech, particularly those of the face, mouth, and larynx, is facilitated by the relaxation of the large voluntary muscles mentioned above. However, there are additional procedures that can be used to aid the speaking act and to restore impaired function. One aspect of the Jacobson procedure is called "differential relaxation," in which specific localized areas of muscle contraction are recognized and modified. For example, exaggeration and release of a persistent frown, or of tension in muscles around the mouth, or of clenched teeth, will aid the speaking process. The muscles of the larynx can be relaxed indirectly by purposely speaking quietly, by using a slightly breathy voice, and by intentionally practicing variation of pitch while speaking. Excessive contraction in the muscles of the neck is often related to posture and may be brought to consciousness by exaggerated positions and attention to the postural abnormalities.

A procedure described in the literature as the "chewing method" can also reduce excessive muscle contraction in the muscles of mastication, the tongue, the pharynx, and the larynx (*14* and *35*). The effectiveness of the method derives from an emphasis on chewing type movements in the production of speech. The chewing movements are less complex than those used in speaking, and by overriding the ordinary speech adjustments they reduce the habitual patterns of hypertension that may have been established.

RELAXATION AND EMOTIONAL STATES. It is a generally recognized fact that anxiety, worry, anger, and related emotional states are often reflected in excessive muscular contraction throughout the body and particularly in the vocal organs. These emotional conditions, when chronic, are detrimental to voice because they create excessive muscle tension. It follows that an attempt to relax specific muscles without attention to emotional states is generally unsuccessful. Consequently, an important phase of vocal reeducation is instruction of the patient in the management of his emotional reactions. This type of therapy may be critically, even vitally, important with the person whose vocal disorder follows treatment for cancer, or where environmental pressures generate chronic detrimental emotional responses. A few suggestions toward this objective can be found in the discussion of mental hygiene that is presented subsequently.

RELAXATION AND THE CLINICIAN. The preceding comments about relaxation have been directed toward the individual who has a voice disorder. It is equally important to stress the importance of relaxation in the clinician. In face to face meetings where therapist-client relationships exist, the former is responsible for the psychological environment as well as the physical setting. The attitudes, emotions, health, and poise of the clinician are revealed subtly and subliminally to the patient through muscle tension, voice, and general behavior. If the therapist is hypertense, the patient frequently acquires a similar condition; conversely, a relaxed, poised clinician tends to create a relaxed state in his patient. It is almost axiomatic that the clinician who cannot achieve complete control of his own emotional states and behavior in the therapist-client situation is not ready for independent professional practice in the field. It is abundantly clear that the hypertense clinician will find it almost impossible to teach a client to relax.

Rationale for Training Listening Skills

Learning to listen, as used here, means the development by the patient of the capacity to distinguish differences in pitch, loudness, quality, and other elements of speech, particularly in his own voice. Some persons hear acutely, yet have difficulty recognizing differences between the pitches of two sounds; others are unable to detect certain changes in loudness; and many cannot distinguish the quality or character of one sound from that of another. It is presumed that persons with one or more of these perceptual deficiencies have a greater tendency toward voice disorders, and, conversely, that they will be able to regulate their voices more efficiently if they develop the ability to recognize the elements of sound in their own voices. It is also presumed that this ability to perceive more completely can be learned and that the individual can then modify his own voice as he monitors his speaking.

The training in listening that has been described above encompasses more than auditory phenomena. When an individual listens to his own voice and attempts to modify it to satisfy an auditory concept, he concurrently makes many subtle adjustments in both muscles and joints within the phonating and resonating systems. The resulting kinesthetic and proprioceptive sensations are amalgamated with the auditory sensations to form complex patterns of adjustment, that is, habit patterns.

Individuals having organically based voice disorders must develop their listening and monitoring skills maximally to enable them to achieve the best possible vocal results at all times. These patients have the task of acquiring audible concepts of their voices, which, although they may be different from normal voices, represent the goal of the best vocal sound that can be produced by their altered vocal organs. Without such a clear goal their practice efforts tend to be aimless and wasteful.

Methods and Procedures for Developing Listening Skill

Improvement of listening skill can be achieved through two routes: (1) systematic comparison and contrast of sounds in order to recognize differences in pitch, loudness, and quality; and (2) focal listening to music and speaking, to separate out particular features of the sounds. In the former when the individual cannot differentiate between two selected pitches, other pairs of sounds with progressively larger intervals should be presented until the fact of difference is noted and the higher and lower elements recognized. The speech clinician should remember that pitch discrimination is influenced by the relative loudness of sounds; consequently, the record player or other sound source should be regulated consistently during both diagnosis and therapy. Comparison and contrast can also be applied to quality differentiation in voice samples, such as hoarse voice and normal voice, hypernasal voice and denasal voice, or in instrumental sounds such as those of the violin and trumpet. Where gross contrasts of the types suggested are not necessary, the pitch, loudness, and quality differences should be reduced progressively.

Focal listening refers to attending to recordings of two or more instruments, consistent with the ability of the patient, in order to hear one instrument within the complex. The same procedure can be applied to the mixure of voices produced by groups of speakers and also to separate vocal elements within a single voice.

41   A number of practical suggestions about ear training are made by Fisher (32:33–6).

These skills in listening represent in some measure the capacity to attend to certain features of sound and to exclude others. The ability may not develop easily or quickly. Practice ordinarily should not be prolonged in any therapy session to the point of fatigue, yet the individual should be encouraged to practice frequently as he hears sounds and voices on the street, on the radio and on television, and in daily conversations. Perceptive listening is part of voice therapy, which is an "all day-every day" process.

Rationale for Regulation of the Breath Pressure

The muscles of the thorax and abdomen that cause exhalation supply the force that causes the vocal cords to vibrate. Optimum phonation occurs when the glottal resistance and breath pressure are adjusted to minimal limits that permit the production of a vocal sound at the desired loudness, pitch, and quality. Vocal training for both singing and normal speaking is basically the acquisition of this optimum balance between vibratory variation in glottal closure and the air pressure that causes the vibration. When a phonatory defect exists, the control of exhalation may be even more important in reeducation of the voice than it is in the training of the normal voice for aesthetic or extensive use.

The inclusion of training in the control of the breath stream as a part of voice therapy is based on the assumptions that some voice disorders are caused by or are related in a secondary way to insufficient breath pressure, to irregular breath flow, or to inadequate breath supply. Training in breath control also presumes that regulation of the stream may compensate for organic problems in the larynx and thereby produce the best vocal sound possible.

Methods and Procedures

Training in control, or regulation of exhalation as used in this presentation, does not refer to deep breathing exercises or blowing or similar respiratory gymnastics. Instead, the term means increased efficiency of breath usage. This improvement can be accomplished indirectly through such exercises as sustaining sung tones for progressively longer periods, humming of musical scales with attention to prolongation of sounds, reading of progressively longer phrases on a single exhalation, and, in general, learning to avoid the wastage of air.

The suggestions about breathing that have just been made are often fundamental to the improvement of phonation when organic disorders such as paralysis and surgical modifications are present in the larynx. If the glottis cannot close adequately during the vibratory cycle, the voice usually has a breathy quality that may be much more prominent than it needs to be. The patient often exhales vigorously in an attempt to produce a loud voice when persons exhibit difficulty understanding him. Under these circumstances the breath noise becomes excessively prominent and tends to obscure what the individual is attempting to say. When these patients learn to reduce the breath pressure and concurrently to increase the precision of their articulatory movements, their speaking is much more intelligible.

The adjustment of breath usage in unilateral laryngeal paralysis and similar glottal problems also helps patients to eliminate dizziness that frequently accompanies their speaking. These individuals often exert excessive respiratory effort in an attempt to compensate for their impaired larynges and consequently over-aerate themselves and become dizzy. Explaining the problem and teaching them to speak with less respiratory effort usually eliminates the discomfort and improves their speech.

Rationale for Attention to Posture

It is unlikely that poor posture in itself causes voice disorders, but it is an important element in voice therapy. Poor posture, as used here, refers especially to that familiar body stance in which the head and neck extend forward, the chest is sunken, and the abdomen protrudes in association with a forward curvature of the lumbar region of the spinal column. The pattern is often described as a combination of kyphosis and lordosis. Posture of this type frequently implies low energy levels and generally inadequate health and physical habits of the patient; it may also reflect his occupation and mode of living.

The person with continuously poor posture may be chronically fatigued or ill. His voice disorder and his posture may represent different aspects of some underlying problem that will not be improved by remedial attention to either voice or posture. On the other hand, poor posture may represent sedentary work and living patterns that produce the undesirable posture just described. Individuals beyond the age of 40 whose occupations cause them to sit almost continuously and who get little or no exercise when they are away from their work will acquire weak muscles that perpetuate the postural faults. Sometimes these individuals are considered to be lazy, which usually is not an accurate assessment of their general debility. However, it should be noted that some individuals are indeed lazy; they may have excellent health but do not have sufficient motivation to maintain adequate posture.

42   How does Fisher associate posture and breathing in a program of
      voice improvement (32:53–8)?

Poor posture affects voice most directly through its interference with the respiratory movements and the associated regulation of breath pressure. The consequences of this problem were sketched in the preceding section. Interference with adequate respiration also causes insufficient aeration of the blood and subsequent fatigue. Reversing the cycle by establishing more adequate respiration will increase the tonus of all muscles and reduce the chronic fatigue.

Poor posture may also create imbalance in the laryngeal musculature and thereby contribute to phonatory disorders. When organic abnormalities are present, the additional burden caused by poor posture increases the difficulties of vocal rehabilitation.

Remedial Procedures

Modification of postural habits may be accomplished, when an underlying physical disorder is not present, by enrolling the patient in a physical education program and requesting the director to help particularly with posture. In addition, the patient should be instructed to perform a series of stretching, bending, and toning calisthenics before breakfast every day. He should also be urged to study his work habits, to vary his posture, to stand and move around at intervals, and to perform isotonic exercises at his desk. He should be encouraged to maintain good posture as a general habit. It has been said that "the best exercise for good posture is good posture."

Rationale for Attention to Physical Hygiene

The preceding considerations of breathing and posture included much that might be considered to be physical hygiene. Elaboration of the subject here to include attention to diet, rest, exercise, smoking, medical care, and dental care is to emphasize the responsibility of the speech pathologist to recognize the need for the total well-being of the patient. The voice is a sensitive indicator of the patient's total physical condition, and the speech pathologist who limits his concern to the larynx and voice is inviting failure.

Extensive recommendations regarding diet, medical attention, and dental care are prescribed, of course, by the appropriate professional personnel, but the speech pathologist can stress the need for adequate food and rest, the benefit of proper exercise, and the detrimental effects of smoking as bases for vocal rehabilitation.

Rationale for Attention to Mental Hygiene

The principles of healthful living that are encompassed within the concept of *physical* hygiene are paralleled by the idea of *mental* hygiene. When a person contracts a disease, he needs the treatment of a physician, but when he is not ill, his everyday health is maintained or improved by practicing the well known principles of hygiene. Similarly, if a person becomes mentally ill, he also needs the therapeutic assistance of those who are professionally trained. However, most persons manage their emotional reactions adequately, communicate satisfactorily with others, and generally have good mental health. Conversely, there are those who experience emotional turmoil; they worry, have anxieties, become angry easily, feel rejected, and find it difficult to communicate with others because they have only limited knowledge of the means of maintaining good mental health. Frequently, these stresses are reflected in excessive muscle contraction or poorly coordinated behavior patterns that affect voice and speech. When organically based vocal problems exist, the effects of undesirable muscular activity are apt to be exaggerated to the further detriment of voice.

Remedial Procedures in Mental Hygiene

There are many kinds of mental hygiene techniques that apply to the individual, the family, and the community, with which the speech pathologist is obligated to be familiar. Mental health is basic in voice therapy, regardless of the origin of the patient's vocal problem. Mental health is also basic in the clinician who directs the therapy.

Fortunately, modification and control of chronic worry, anxiety, anger, and similar emotional responses are possible, as are other forms of behavior. Many patterns of response exist because they were learned. The child who grows up in an environment where parents' reactions are volatile and violent in response to problems and crises accepts such behavior as the expected or normal response. To be normal in his group he behaves as do his associates. Similarly, withdrawal, lack of communication, insulting remarks, and other reactions to frustration and inadequacy are accepted and perpetuated. While many of these behavior patterns begin in childhood, it must be realized that they may also develop later as the individual attempts to adapt to his living and work situations. Usually the person finds his responses to be satisfactory to himself; they are, from his limited viewpoint, the best means of coping with his problems. He accepts his responses and obtains a certain degree of comfort, or even pleasure, from them. The importance of the attitudes that he may not recognize objectively, or that he does not admit, becomes evident in their tenacious resistance to change. The contributions of these various forms of behavior to voice problems are accomplished through excessive muscle tensions, poor posture, and reluctance to admit a need for vocal change. Such behavior patterns and attitudes are related to mental health and hygiene; they are a concern of the speech pathologist.

The preceding sketch, of course, oversimplifies the behavior related to unhealthy attitudes and emotional response. It does not dwell on the fact that the reactions of some individuals to certain life situations are neither reflections of early environment nor inadequate adjustment to social and economic problems; nor does it point out that atypical reactions sometimes represent successful on-going struggles with clearly recognized problems. The earlier comments also do not include the fact that emotions and the behavioral responses to them often have a glandular or other biochemical base.

The modification and management of a learned response begins with an analysis or study of that response. The speech pathologist will benefit from a week-long program for himself, in which he describes in writing his own response to occurrences that caused an emotional reaction. He will find such an exercise to be insightful and useful in assessing his own emotional behavior and even more helpful in guiding his patients who have voice disorders.

The first step in the study of emotional response is observation and description. The clinician should note each of his own reactions, including both the feelings that he experiences and his overt behavior. Next he should judge the adequacy or appropriateness of his response and consider what other responses he could have made in the particular circumstances. To assess adequacy and appropriateness it is necessary for the individual to appraise not only the interpersonal factors but also his own physical condition and mental attitudes at the time of his emotional episode. The individual who is ill, fatigued, or beset with the anxiety of facing a crisis is likely to perceive, interpret, and react quite differently from the way he would have responded had the impinging factors not been present. The clinician may discover that some of his own responses could have been more appropriate and consequently should have been different; he may also recognize that he is unwilling to change his behavior because it gives him some sort of satisfaction. He may rationalize his remarks or other reactions on the basis of being "honest" or "helpful," while, in fact, he is attempting to justify inadequate consideration of the other person's condition or situation. If he, a professional worker, can have such attitudes and reactions, he should realize that his patients can also have them and, furthermore, that such behavior can influence the rehabilitative process.

The individual who has a voice problem that is related to disease or surgical intervention may have genuine concerns about his life expectancy, his job, and his association with others. These considerations may adversely influence his voice and his vocal rehabilitation, and they certainly must be recognized and managed considerately and honestly in therapy but without interference with it. Occasionally, a patient may be so discouraged or depressed that he cannot respond to voice therapy and its infused mental health assistance. That person is a candidate for therapy by a psychiatrist or clinical psychologist, either in an independent program or in one that combines mental health training and vocal rehabilitation. The speech pathologist has the ethical responsibility to make appropriate referrals when indicated and to carry his full share of the rehabilitation program.

SUMMARY OF VOCAL THERAPY FOR ORGANIC VOICE DISORDERS

There are several types of therapy available to the individual who has an organically based voice disorder. The selection of remedial procedures and their effectiveness will be determined by the etiology of the disorder, the art and skill of those conducting the therapy, and the cooperation of the patient. The foregoing statement emphasizes the fact that therapy is individualized and that the therapist selects from among the many possible procedures to develop a specific rehabilitative program. ᘏᘏᘏ

bibliography

1. Arnold, G. E., "Vocal Nodules and Polyps: Laryngeal Tissue Reaction to Habitual Hyperkinetic Dysphonia," *Journal of Speech and Hearing Disorders,* 27 (1962), 205–17.
2. ———, "Vocal Rehabilitation of Paralytic Dysphonia. X. Functional Results of Intrachordal Injection," *Archives of Otolaryngology,* 78, No. 2 (1963), 179–86.
3. Aronson, A. E., Joe R. Brown, Edward M. Litin, and John S. Pearson, "Spastic Dysphonia. I. Neurologic and Psychiatric Aspects," *Journal of Speech and Hearing Disorders,* 33 (1968), 203–17.
4. ———, "Spastic Dysphonia. II. Comparison with Essential (Voice) Tremor and Other Neurologic and Psychogenic Dysphonias," *Journal of Speech and Hearing Disorders,* 33 (1968), 219–31.
5. Ash, J. E., "Pathologic and Epithelial Changes and Tumors of the Larynx," Chapter 7 in *Voice and Speech Disorders: Medical Aspects,* Nathaniel M. Levin, ed. (Springfield, Illinois: Charles C Thomas, Publisher, 1962).
6. Ballenger, Howard Charles, and John J. Ballenger, *A Manual of Otology, Rhinology and Laryngology,* 4th ed. (Philadelphia: Lea & Febiger, 1954).
7. ———, *Diseases of the Nose, Throat and Ear,* 10th ed. (Philadelphia: Lea & Febiger, 1957).
8. Ballenger, John Jacob, and Contributors, *Diseases of the Nose, Throat and Ear,* 11th ed. (Philadelphia: Lea & Febiger, 1969).

9. Baker, D. C., "Contact Ulcer of the Larynx," *The Laryngoscope,* 64 (1954), 73–8.

10. Beranek, L. L., *Acoustic Measurements* (New York: John Wiley & Sons, Inc., 1949).

11. Brodnitz, Friedrich S., "Vocal Rehabilitation," *American Academy of Ophthalmology and Otolaryngology* (Section on Instruction—Home Study Courses) (Chicago: An American Medical Association Publication, 1959).

12. ———, "Contact Ulcer of the Larynx," *Archives of Otolaryngology,* 74 (1961), 70–80.

13. ———, "Goals, Results and Limitations of Vocal Rehabilitation," *Archives of Otolaryngology,* 77 (1963), 148–56.

14. ———, and E. Froeschels, "Treatment of Nodules of Vocal Cords by the Chewing Method," *Archives of Otolaryngology,* 60 (1954), 560–65.

15. Brown, Joe R., and Josephine Simonson, "Organic Voice Tremor," *Neurology,* 13 (1963), 520–25.

16. Butler, R. Melvin, and Fritz H. Moser, "The Padded Dash Syndrome: Blunt Trauma to the Larynx and Trachea," *The Laryngoscope,* 78, No. 7 (1968), 1172–82.

17. Cooper, Morton, and Alan M. Nahum, "Vocal Rehabilitation for Contact Ulcer of the Larynx," *Archives of Otolaryngology,* 85 (1967), 41–6.

18. Damsté, P. H., "Virilization of the Voice Due to Anabolic Steroids," *Folia Phoniatrica,* 16 (1964), 10–18.

19. ———, "Voice Change in Adult Women Caused by Virilizing Agents," *Journal of Speech and Hearing Disorders,* 32 (1967), 126–32.

20. Daly, John F., "The Hoarse Patient," *Postgraduate Medicine,* 34 (1963), 488–92.

21. Darley, Frederic L., *Diagnosis and Appraisal of Communication Disorders* (Englewood Cliffs, New Jersey: Prentice-Hall, Inc., 1964).

22. Davis, D. S., and D. R. Boone, "Pitch Discrimination and Tonal Memory Abilities in Adult Voice Patients," *Journal of Speech and Hearing Disorders,* 10 (1967), 811–15.

23. Devine, Kenneth D., "Laryngectomy," *Archives of Otolaryngology,* 78 (1963), 816–25.

24. DeWeese, David D., and William H. Saunders, *Textbook of Otolaryngology,* 2nd ed. (St. Louis: C. V. Mosby Company, 1964).

25. Diedrich, William M., and K. A. Youngstrom, *Alaryngeal Speech* (Springfield, Illinois: Charles C Thomas, Publisher, 1966).

26. Dolowitz, David D., *Basic Otolaryngology* (New York: The Blakiston Division, McGraw-Hill Book Company, 1964).

27. *Dorland's Illustrated Medical Dictionary,* 23rd ed. (Philadelphia: The W. B. Saunders Company, 1957).

28. Eisenson, Jon, Schulamith Kastein, and Norma Schneiderman, "An Investigation into the Ability of Voice Defectives to Discriminate Among Differences in Pitch and Loudness," *Journal of Speech and Hearing Disorders,* 23 (1958), 577–82.

29. *Encyclopaedia Britannica, Inc.* (Chicago: William Benton, Publisher, 1966).

30. Faaborg-Anderson, K., "Electromyographic Investigation of Intrinsic Laryngeal Muscles in Humans," *Acta Physiologica Scandinavica,* Supplement, 140 (1957), 1–148.

31. ————, and A. M. Jensen, "Unilateral Paralysis of the Superior Laryngeal Nerve," *Acta Oto-laryngologica,* 57 (1964), 155–59.

32. Fisher, Hilda B., *Improving Voice and Articulation* (Boston: Houghton Mifflin Company, 1966).

33. Flanagan, J. L., "Some Properties of the Glottal Sound Source," *Journal of Speech and Hearing Research,* 1 (1958), 99–116.

34. Frable, M. A. S., "Hoarseness, a Symptom of Premenstrual Tension," *Archives of Otolaryngology,* 75 (1962), 66–8.

35. Froeschels, Emil, "Chewing Method as Therapy," *Archives of Otolaryngology,* 56 (1952), 427–34.

36. Gardner, Warren H., "Adjustment Problems of Laryngectomized Women," *Archives of Otolaryngology,* 83 (1966), 31–42.

37. Gargan, William, *Why Me?* (New York: Doubleday and Company, 1969).

38. Gray, Henry, *Anatomy of the Human Body,* 27th ed. (Philadelphia: Lea & Febiger, 1959).

39. Greene, Margaret C. L., *The Voice and Its Disorders,* 2nd ed. (Philadelphia: J. B. Lippincott Company, 1964).

40. Hagan, P. J., "Vocal Cord Paralysis," *Annals of Otology, Rhinology and Laryngology,* 72 (1963), 206–22.

41. Harned, Je, *Medical Terminology Made Easy* (Chicago: Physicians' Record Company, 1951).

42. Holinger, P. H., K. C. Johnston, and R. J. McMahon, "Hoarseness in Infants and Children," *Eye, Ear, Nose and Throat Monographs,* 31 (1952), 247–51.

43. ————, and K. C. Johnston, "Contact Ulcer of the Larynx," *Journal of the American Medical Association,* 1122 (1960), 511–15.

44. Hollien, H., and R. W. Wendahl, "Perceptual Study of Vocal Fry," *Journal of the Acoustical Society of America,* 43 (1968), 506–9.

45. Jackson, C., "Contact Ulcer of the Larynx," *Annals of Otology, Rhinology and Laryngology,* 37 (1928), 227–30.

46. ————, and C. L. Jackson, *The Larynx and Its Diseases* (Philadelphia: The W. B. Saunders Company, 1937).

47. ————, *Diseases and Injuries of the Larynx* (New York: The Macmillan Company, 1942).

48. ————, *Diseases of the Nose, Throat and Ear* (Philadelphia: The W. B. Saunders Company, 1959).

49. Jacobson, Edmund, *You Must Relax* (New York: McGraw-Hill Book Company, 1934).

50. ————, *Progressive Relaxation* (Chicago: University of Chicago Press, 1938).

51. Johnson, W., S. F. Brown, J. F. Curtis, C. W. Edney, and J. Keaster, *Speech Handicapped School Children* (New York: Harper & Row, Publishers, 1956).

52. Johnson, Wendell, Frederic Darley, and D. C. Spriestersbach, *Diagnostic Methods in Speech Pathology* (New York: Harper & Row, Publishers, 1963).

53. Konig, W. F., and H. von Leden, "The Peripheral Nervous System of the Human Larynx. III. The Development," *Archives of Otolaryngology*, 74 (1961), 494–500.

54. Lauder, Edmond, "The Role of the Laryngectomee in Post-Laryngectomy Voice Instruction," *Journal of Speech and Hearing Disorders*, 30 (1965), 145–57.

55. Lederer, Francis L., *Diseases of the Ear, Nose and Throat*, 3rd ed. (Philadelphia: F. A. Davis Company, 1942).

56. Levin, Nathaniel M. ed., *Voice and Speech Disorders: Medical Aspects* (Springfield, Illinois: Charles C Thomas, Publisher, 1962).

57. Lieberman, Philip, "Vocal Cord Motion in Man," *Annals of the New York Academy of Sciences*, 155 (1968), 28–38.

58. Luchsinger, Richard, and Godfrey E. Arnold, *Voice–Speech–Language* (Belmont, California: Wadsworth Publishing Company, 1965).

59. Luse, Eleanor M., *A Study of Vocal Structures and Speech in Relation to Metabolic Rate* (Northwestern University: Unpublished Dissertation, 1948).

60. Mårtensson, A., "The Functional Organization of the Intrinsic Laryngeal Muscles," *Annals of the New York Academy of Science*, 155 (1968), 91–6.

61. McWilliams, B. J., and R. H. Musgrave, "Differential Diagnosis and Management of Hypernasal Voices in Children," *Transactions of the American Academy of Ophthalmology and Otolaryngology*, 69 (1965), 322–31.

62. Milisen, Robert, "Method of Evaluation and Diagnosis of Speech Disorders," *Handbook of Speech Pathology*, Lee Edward Travis, ed. (New York: Appleton-Century-Crofts, Inc., 1957).

63. ———, "Methods of Evaluation and Diagnosis of Speech Disorders," *Handbook of Speech Pathology and Audiology*, Lee Edward Travis, ed. (New York: Appleton-Century-Crofts, Inc., 1971).

64. Miller, Alden, "First Experiences with the Asai Technique for Vocal Rehabilitation after Total Laryngectomy," *Annals of Otology, Rhinology and Laryngology*, 76 (1967), 829.

65. Moore, Paul, "Otolaryngology and Speech Pathology," *The Laryngoscope*, 78 (1968), 1500–9.

66. ———, "Discussion of the Preceding Paper," *Annals of the New York Academy of Sciences*, 155 (1968), 39–40.

67. ———, "Voice Disorders Organically Based," *Handbook of Speech Pathology and Audiology*, Lee Edward Travis, ed. (New York: Appleton-Century-Crofts, Inc., 1971).

68. Moore, Paul, and Hans von Leden, "Dynamic Variations of the Vibratory Pattern in the Normal Larynx," *Folia Phoniatrica*, 10 (1958), 205–38.

69. ———, Frazer D. White, and Hans von Leden, "Ultra-High Speed Photography in Laryngeal Physiology," *Journal of Speech and Hearing Disorders*, 27 (1962), 165–71.

70. ———, and Thomas B. Abbott, "Defects of Speech," Chapter 38 in John J. Ballenger, *Diseases of the Nose, Throat and Ear*, 11th ed. (Philadelphia: Lea & Febiger, Publisher, 1969).

71. Murphy, Albert T., *Functional Voice Disorders* (Englewood Cliffs, New Jersey: Prentice-Hall, Inc., 1965).

72. Myerson, Mervin C., *The Human Larynx* (Springfield, Illinois: Charles C Thomas, Publisher, 1964).

73. O'Neill, J. J., and J. A. McGee, "Management of Benign Tumors in Children, Preoperative, Operative and Postoperative," *Annals of Otology, Rhinology and Laryngology*, 71 (1962), 480–88.

74. Peacher, Georgiana M., "Vocal Therapy for Contact Ulcer of the Larynx, A Follow-up of Seventy Patients," *The Laryngoscope*, 71 (1961), 37–47.

75. ———, and P. Holinger, "Contact Ulcer of the Larynx. The Role of Vocal Re-education," *Archives of Otolaryngology*, 46 (1947), 617–23.

76. Poe, D. L., and P. Seager, "Congenital Laryngeal Web: Its Eradication," *Archives of Otolaryngology*, 47 (1948), 46–8.

77. Ptacek, P. H., and E. K. Sander, "Maximum Duration of Phonation," *Journal of Speech and Hearing Disorders*, 28 (1963), 171–82.

78. Robe, E. Y., Paul Moore, A. H. Andrews, Jr., and P. H. Holinger, "A Study of the Role of Certain Factors in the Development of Speech after Laryngectomy: Part I. Type of Operation; Part II. Site of Pseudoglottis; Part III. Coordination of Speech with Respiration," *The Laryngoscope*, 66 (1956), 173–86; 382–401; 481–99.

79. ———, K. Brumlik, and P. Moore, "A Study of Spastic Dysphonia: Neurologic and Electroencephalographic Abnormalities," *The Laryngoscope*, 70 (1960), 219–45.

80. Senturia, Ben H., and Frank B. Wilson, "Otorhinolaryngic Findings in Children with Voice Disorders," *Annals of Otology, Rhinology and Laryngology*, 77 (1968), 1027–42.

81. Shearer, William M., *Illustrated Speech Anatomy*, 2nd ed. (Springfield, Illinois: Charles C Thomas, Publisher, 1968).

82. Sherman, D. H., "The Merits of Backward Playing of Connected Speech in the Scaling of Voice Quality Disorders," *Journal of Speech and Hearing Disorders*, 19 (1954), 312–21.

83. Snidecor, John C. and others, *Speech Rehabilitation of the Laryngectomized* (Springfield, Illinois: Charles C Thomas, Publisher, 1962).

84. *Stedman's Medical Dictionary*, 21st ed. (Baltimore: Williams and Wilkins, Publisher, 1966).

85. Sullivan, W. W., M. E. Sauer, and G. Corssen, "A Study of the

Rotary Component of the Motion of the Arytenoid Cartilage in Man,"
Texas Reports of Biology and Medicine, 18 (1960), 284–87.

86. van den Berg, Janwillem, "Myoelastic-aerodynamic Theory of Voice
Production," *Journal of Speech and Hearing Research,* 1 (1958),
227–43.

87. Van Riper, Charles, *Principles and Practice of Speech Correction,*
4th ed. (Englewood Cliffs, New Jersey: Prentice-Hall, Inc., 1963).

88. ———, and John V. Irwin, *Voice and Articulation* (Englewood Cliffs,
New Jersey: Prentice-Hall, Inc., 1958).

89. von Leden, Hans, and Paul Moore, "Contact Ulcer of the Larynx:
Experimental Observations," *Archives of Otolaryngology,* 72 (1960),
746–52.

90. ———, "The Mechanics of the Crico-arytenoid Joint," *Archives of
Otolaryngology,* 73 (1961), 541–50.

91. ———, "Vibratory Pattern of the Vocal Cords in Unilateral Laryngeal Paralysis," *Acta Oto-laryngologica,* 53 (1961), 493–506.

92. Ward, Paul H., Jay W. Sanders, Ronald Goldman, and G. Paul
Moore, "Diplophonia," *Annals of Otology, Rhinology and Laryngology,* 78 (1969), 771–75.

93. Wendahl, R. W., "Some Parameters of Auditory Roughness," *Folia
Phoniatrica,* 18 (1966), 26–32.

94. West, Robert, Merle Ansberry, and Anna Carr, *The Rehabilitation
of Speech,* 3rd ed. (New York: Harper and Row, Publisher, 1957).

95. ———, and Merle Ansberry, *The Rehabilitation of Speech,* 4th ed.
(New York: Harper and Row, Publisher, 1968).

96. Wilson, D. Kenneth, "Voice Re-education in Benign Laryngeal Pathology," *Eye, Ear, Nose and Throat Monthly,* 45 (1966), 76–80.

97. Wood, Kenneth Scott, "Terminology and Nomenclature," *Handbook
of Speech Pathology,* Lee Edward Travis, ed. (New York: Appleton-
Century-Crofts, Inc., 1957).

index